Disorders and Treatment of the Cerebral Venous System

Editor

SHAHID M. NIMJEE

NEUROSURGERY
CLINICS OF NORTH AMERICA

www.neurosurgery.theclinics.com

Consulting Editors
RUSSELL R. LONSER
DANIEL K. RESNICK

July 2024 • Volume 35 • Number 3

ELSEVIER

1600 John F. Kennedy Boulevard • Suite 1800 • Philadelphia, Pennsylvania, 19103-2899

http://www.theclinics.com

NEUROSURGERY CLINICS OF NORTH AMERICA Volume 35, Number 3
July 2024 ISSN 1042-3680, ISBN-13: 978-0-443-24640-1

Editor: Stacy Eastman
Developmental Editor: Akshay Samson

Neurosurgery Clinics of North America (ISSN 1042-3680) is published quarterly by Elsevier Inc., 360 Park Avenue South, New York, NY 10010-1710. Months of issue are January, April, July, and October. Business and Editorial Offices: 1600 John F. Kennedy Blvd., Suite 1800, Philadelphia, PA 19103-2899. Customer Service Office: 11830 Westline Industrial Drive, St. Louis, MO 63146. Periodicals postage paid at New York, NY, and additional mailing offices. Subscription prices are $465.00 per year (US individuals), $499.00 per year (Canadian individuals), $579.00 per year (international individuals), $100.00 per year (US students), $255.00 per year (international students), and $100.00 per year (Canadian students). For institutional access pricing please contact Customer Service via the contact information below. International air speed delivery is included in all *Clinics* subscription prices. All prices are subject to change without notice. **POSTMASTER:** Send address changes to *Neurosurgery Clinics of North America*, Elsevier Periodicals Customer Service, 11830 Westline Industrial Drive, St. Louis, MO 63146. **Customer Service: 1-800-654-2452 (US and Canada). From outside the US and Canada, call: 1-314-453-7041. Fax: 1-314-453-5170. E-mail: JournalsCustomerService-usa@elsevier.com (for print support) and journalsonlinesupport-usa@elsevier.com (for online support).**

Reprints. For copies of 100 or more, of articles in this publication, please contact the Commercial Reprints Department, Elsevier Inc., 360 Park Avenue South, New York, NY 10010-1710. Tel. 212-633-3874; Fax: 212-633-3820; E-mail: reprints@elsevier.com.

Neurosurgery Clinics of North America is covered in *MEDLINE/PubMed (Index Medicus), EMBASE/Excerpta Medica, and Current Contents/Clinical Medicine (CC/CM)*.

Contributors

CONSULTING EDITORS

RUSSELL R. LONSER, MD
Professor and Chair, Department of
Neurological Surgery, The Ohio State
University Wexner Medical Center, Columbus,
Ohio

DANIEL K. RESNICK, MD, MS
Professor and Vice Chairman, Program
Director, Department of Neurosurgery,
University of Wisconsin-Madison School of
Medicine and Public Health, Madison,
Wisconsin

EDITOR

SHAHID M. NIMJEE, MD, PhD
Professor and Vice Chair, Department of
Neurosurgery, The Ohio State University
Wexner Medical Center, Columbus, Ohio

AUTHORS

MATTHEW ANDERSON, MD
Acting Instructor, Department of Neurological
Surgery, University of Washington, Seattle,
Washington

ELIZA BAIRD-DANIEL, MD
Resident Physician, Department of
Neurological Surgery, University of
Washington, Seattle, Washington

DANIEL L. BARROW, MD
Pamela Rollins Professor and Chairman,
Department of Neurosurgery, Emory
University School of Medicine, Atlanta,
Georgia

BRANDON M. BENEDUCE, BS
CereVasc Inc., Charlestown, Massachusetts

ALEJANDRO BERENSTEIN, MD
Professor, Department of Neurosurgery, Icahn
School of Medicine at Mount Sinai, New York,
New York

MEHDI BOUSLAMA, MD, MSc
Fellow, Department of Neurosurgery, Jacobs
School of Medicine and Biomedical Sciences,
University at Buffalo, Buffalo, New York

WALEED BRINJIKJI, MD
Professor, Departments of Radiology and
Neurosurgery, Mayo Clinic, Rochester,
Minnesota

CHARLOTTE CHUNG, MD, PhD
Fellow, Departments of Radiology and
Neurosurgery, NYU Langone Health, Bellevue
Hospital Center, New York, New York

JONATHAN DALLAS, MD
Neurosurgery Resident, Department of
Neurosurgery, University of Southern
California, Los Angeles, California

BADIH J. DAOU, MD
Neurosurgery Fellow, Department of
Neurosurgery, Barrow Neurological Institute,
St. Joseph's Hospital and Medical Center,
Phoenix, Arizona

JASON M. DAVIES, MD, PhD
Associate Professor, Departments of
Neurosurgery and Bioinformatics, Jacobs
School of Medicine and Biomedical Sciences,
Canon Stroke and Vascular Research Center,
University at Buffalo, Jacobs Institute, Buffalo,
New York

ALEXANDRA N. DEMETRIOU, MA
Medical Student, Department of Neurosurgery, University of Southern California, Los Angeles, California

ALEX DEVARAJAN, BS
Medical Student, Department of Neurosurgery, Icahn School of Medicine at Mount Sinai, New York, New York

ANDREW F. DUCRUET, MD
Associate Professor, Department of Neurosurgery, Barrow Neurological Institute, St. Joseph's Hospital and Medical Center, Phoenix, Arizona

KAREEM EL NAAMANI, MD
Postdoctoral Research Fellow, Department of Neurological Surgery, Thomas Jefferson University Hospital, Philadelphia, Pennsylvania

JOHANNA T. FIFI, MD
Professor, Department of Neurosurgery, Icahn School of Medicine at Mount Sinai, New York, New York

DARYL GOLDMAN, MD
Resident, Department of Neurosurgery, Icahn School of Medicine at Mount Sinai, New York, New York

MICHAEL REID GOOCH, MD
Assistant Professor, Department of Neurological Surgery, Thomas Jefferson University Hospital, Philadelphia, Pennsylvania

BRADLEY A. GROSS, MD
Associate Professor, Department of Neurological Surgery, University of Pittsburgh Medical Center, University of Pittsburgh School of Medicine, Pittsburgh, Pennsylvania

JONATHAN A. GROSSBERG, MD
Associate Professor, Department of Neurological Surgery, Emory University, Atlanta, Georgia

CARL B. HEILMAN, MD
Chair and Professor, Department of Neurosurgery, Tufts Medical Center, Boston, Massachusetts

STEVEN B. HOUSLEY, MD, MS
Fellow, Department of Neurosurgery, Jacobs School of Medicine and Biomedical Sciences, University at Buffalo, Buffalo, New York

BRIAN M. HOWARD, MD
Associate Professor, Departments of Neurosurgery and, Radiology and Imaging Sciences, Division of Interventional Neuroradiology, Emory University School of Medicine, Atlanta, Georgia

SAMER S. HOZ, MD
Research Fellow, Department of Neurological Surgery, University of Pittsburgh Medical Center, University of Pittsburgh School of Medicine, Pittsburgh, Pennsylvania

PASCAL JABBOUR, MD
Distinguished Professor of Neurological Surgery and Radiology, Chief, Department of Neurological Surgery, Thomas Jefferson University Hospital, Professor of Neurological Surgery, Chief, Division of Neurovascular Surgery and Endovascular Neurosurgery, Thomas Jefferson University Hospital, Philadelphia, Pennsylvania

MICHAEL J. LANG, MD
Assistant Professor, Department of Neurological Surgery, University of Pittsburgh Medical Center, University of Pittsburgh School of Medicine, Pittsburgh, Pennsylvania

MICHAEL R. LEVITT, MD
Professor, Departments of Neurological Surgery, Radiology, Neurology, Mechanical Engineering, and Stroke & Applied Neuroscience Center, University of Washington, Seattle, Washington

LI MA, MD, PhD
Research Fellow, Department of Neurological Surgery, University of Pittsburgh Medical Center, University of Pittsburgh School of Medicine, Pittsburgh, Pennsylvania

WILLIAM J. MACK, MD, MBA
Professor, Department of Neurosurgery, University of Southern California, Los Angeles, California

ADEL M. MALEK, MD, PhD
Professor of Neurosurgery, Director of Cerebrovascular and Endovascular Division, Tufts Medical Center, Boston, MassaChusetts; CereVasc Inc., Charlestown, Massachusetts

MATTHEW J. McPHEETERS, MD, MBA
Fellow, Department of Neurosurgery, Jacobs School of Medicine and Biomedical Sciences, University at Buffalo, Buffalo, New York

RAYMOND MICHAEL MEYER, MD
Acting Instructor, Department of Neurological Surgery, University of Washington, Seattle, Washington

J. MOCCO, MD, MS
Professor and System Vice Chair, Department of Neurological Surgery, Mount Sinai Hospital, New York, New York

PETER KIM NELSON, MD
Radiologist, Department of Radiology and Neurosurgery, NYU Langone Health, Bellevue Hospital Center, New York, New York

VINCENT N. NGUYEN, MD
Vascular Neurosurgery Clinical Fellow, Department of Neurosurgery, University of Southern California, Los Angeles, California

EREZ NOSSEK, MD
Neurosurgeon, Department of Radiology and Neurosurgery, NYU Langone Health, Bellevue Hospital Center, New York, New York

NITESH P. PATEL, MD
Department of Neurosurgery, Mayo Clinic, Rochester, Minnesota

KUNAL P. RAYGOR, MD
Fellow, Department of Neurosurgery, Jacobs School of Medicine and Biomedical Sciences, University at Buffalo, Buffalo, New York

EYTAN RAZ, MD, PhD
Associate Professor, Department of Radiology and Neurosurgery, NYU Langone Health, Bellevue Hospital Center, New York, New York

TYLER SCULLEN, MD
Fellow, Department of Neurosurgery, Jacobs School of Medicine and Biomedical Sciences, University at Buffalo, Buffalo, New York

MAKSIM SHAPIRO, MD
Radiologist, Department of Radiology and Neurosurgery, NYU Langone Health, Bellevue Hospital Center, New York, New York

VERA SHARASHIDZE, MD
Radiologist, Department of Radiology and Neurosurgery, NYU Langone Health, Bellevue Hospital Center, New York, New York

TOMOYOSHI SHIGEMATSU, MD, PhD
Assistant Professor, Department of Neurosurgery, Icahn School of Medicine at Mount Sinai, New York, New York

STAVROPOULA I. TJOUMAKARIS, MD
President Elect Cerebrovascular Section, Department of Neurological Surgery, Thomas Jefferson University Hospital, Philadelphia, Pennsylvania

KURT YAEGER, MD
Assistant Professor, Department of Neurological Surgery, Houston Methodist Hospital, Houston, Texas

Contributors

RAYMOND MICHAEL MEYER, MD
Acting Instructor, Department of Neurological
Surgery, University of Washington, Seattle,
Washington

J. MOCCO, MD, MS
Professor and System Chairman, Department
of Neurological Surgery, Mount Sinai, New York,
New York, New York

PETER KIM NELSON, MD
Neurologist, Department of Radiology and
Neurosurgery, NYU Langone Health, Bellevue
Hospital Center, New York, New York

VINCENT M. TUTINO, MD
Jacobs Research Center, Office of... ...,
Department of ... ... Surgery, University at
Buffalo...

DR. E MONSERS, MD
Department of Neurological Surgery, ...
Neurosurgery, NYU Langone Health, Bellevue
Hospital Center, New York, New York

MAYSAM A. PATEL, MD
Department of Neurosurgery, Mount Sinai
Health, New York

RONALD PRESTON, MD
Fellow, Department of Neurosurgery,
Department of Radiology, Mount Sinai Health,
Department of Neurosurgery, New York, New
York, New York

EYTAN RAZ, MD, PhD
Associate Professor, Department of Radiology
and Neurosurgery, NYU Langone Health,
Bellevue Hospital Center, New York, New York

TYLER SOULLEN, MD
Fellow, Department of Neuroradiology, Jacobs
School of Medicine and Biomedical Sciences,
University at Buffalo, Buffalo, New York

KARISM SHAPIRO, MD
Radiologist, Department of Radiology and
Neurosurgery, NYU Langone Health, Bellevue
Hospital Center, New York, New York

NSR SHARASHIDZE, MD
Assistant Professor, Department of Radiology and
Neurosurgery, NYU Langone Health, Bellevue
Hospital Center, New York, New York

TOMOYOSHI SHOEMATSU, MD, PhD
Fellow, Department of Neurosurgery,
Department of Radiology, Mount Sinai Health,
New York, New York, New York

STAVROPOULA L. TJOUMAKARIS, MD
Associate Professor, Department of Surgery,
Department of Neurosurgery, Thomas
Jefferson University, Philadelphia, Pennsyl-
vania

SUNNY Y. CHO, MD
Neurologist, Department of Department of
Neurosurgery and Neurology, Mount Montreal
Medical Center...

Contents

Cerebrospinal fluid-venous fistulas (CSFVFs) were first described in 2014 and have since become an increasingly diagnosed cause of spontaneous intracranial hypotension due to increased clinical recognition and advancements in diagnostic modalities. In this review, the authors discuss CSFVF epidemiology, the variety of clinical presentations, the authors' preferred diagnostic approach, recent advancements in diagnostic methods, treatment options, current challenges, and directions of future research.

Carotid cavernous fistulae (CCFs) are arteriovenous shunts involving the cavernous sinus. CCFs are defined as direct or indirect. Direct CCFs are treated by deconstructive or reconstructive techniques depending on whether the affected internal carotid artery is required to perfuse the ipsilateral cerebral hemisphere, as determined by a balloon test occlusion. Indirect CCFs, or dural fistulae of the cavernous sinus wall, are most often treated with transvenous embolization. Stereotactic radiosurgery is reserved for cases of indirect CCFs that are not completely obliterated by embolization. Overall, cure rates are high with relatively low complication rates.

Dural arteriovenous fistulas are rare cerebrovascular lesions arising from abnormal connections between an artery and a vein. Though rare, high-grade aggressive lesions can cause hemorrhagic events and non-hemorrhagic neurologic deficits if left untreated. Treatment options vary based on angioarchitecture, location, and patient characteristics and range from conservative observation to palliative treatment, radiosurgery, endovascular embolization, and open surgery. The main goal of treatment is to obliterate flow through the abnormal connection and prevent further arterial flow to the venous system.

Cerebral venous sinus thrombosis (CVST) is a rare type of stroke indicated by the formation of blood clots within the dural venous sinuses. These are large venous conduits that are situated between the 2 layers of the dura mater which are responsible for draining blood from the brain and returning it to the systemic circulation. Cortical venous thrombosis refers to the blockage of veins on the brain's cortical surface. Cerebral venous thrombosis encompasses both dural and cortical vein occlusions.

Developmental venous anomalies (DVAs) are the most common vascular malformation detected on intracranial cross-sectional imaging. They are generally benign lesions thought to drain normal parenchyma. Spontaneous hemorrhages attributed to DVAs are rare and should be ascribed to associated cerebral cavernous malformations, flow-related shunts, or venous outflow obstruction. Contrast-enhanced MRI, susceptibility-weighted imaging, and high-field MRI are ideal tools for visualizing vessel connectivity and associated lesions. DVAs are not generally considered targets for treatment. Preservation of DVAs is an established practice in the microsurgical or radiosurgical treatment of associated lesions.

NEUROSURGERY CLINICS OF NORTH AMERICA

SERIES OF RELATED INTEREST

Neurologic Clinics
https://www.neurologic.theclinics.com/
Neuroimaging Clinics
https://www.neuroimaging.theclinics.com/

THE CLINICS ARE AVAILABLE ONLINE!
Access your subscription at:
www.theclinics.com

Preface

The Venous System of the Central Nervous System: Anatomy, Diseases, Treatments, and Pathway to Innovation

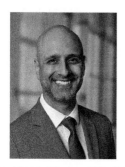

Shahid M. Nimjee, MD, PhD
Editor

It is a privilege to serve as a guest editor for this *Neurosurgery Clinics of North America* issue, focusing on the venous system of the central nervous system (CNS).

As anatomy lays the foundation for what we need to know as neurosurgeons, this issue of *Neurosurgery Clinics of North America* begins with a comprehensive overview of the venous anatomy of the CNS.

The subsequent articles provide in-depth summaries of the diseases of the cerebral venous system, largely the result of thrombosis, infection, stenosis, trauma, and congenital or acquired malformations. Advancements in endovascular technology for the arterial system of the CNS have enabled treatment of venous disease. Many of the catheters and devices initially designed for the arterial system have demonstrated both safety and efficacy in accessing the venous system to diagnose and treat the pathologies described in this issue. Idiopathic intracranial hypertension, once solely treated with ventriculoperitoneal or lumboperitoneal shunting, has seen venous sinus stenting emerge to resolve papilledema effectively. This concept has now been successfully translated into patients who present with pulsatile tinnitus. While the articles on carotid-cavernous fistulas and dural arteriovenous fistulas describe venous embolization as a mainstay of treatment, the article on cerebrospinal fluid–venous fistula describes how venous embolization successfully treats spontaneous intracranial hypotension. The final two articles describe innovative approaches to treating paralysis and hydrocephalus by implanting endovascular devices in the venous sinuses.

I am grateful to the contributors to this issue of *Neurosurgery Clinics of North America*, who are not only leading experts but also pioneers who have developed the diagnostic criteria and treatment paradigms discussed in the following chapters. I hope this issue serves as an accessible

Neurosurg Clin N Am 35 (2024) xi–xii
https://doi.org/10.1016/j.nec.2024.04.001

reference for understanding the anatomy of the cerebral venous system, the venous diseases encountered by neurosurgeons, and the opportunities to potentially change how we approach conditions like paralysis and hydrocephalus by innovatively targeting the venous vasculature.

DISCLOSURES

Dr S.M. Nimjee is co-founder of Basking Biosciences; serves on the Data Safety Monitoring Board for Cerenovus; serves as a speaker for Medtronic, Inc; serves on the Medical Advisory Board for Hyperfine, Inc; and receives grant funding from the National Institutes of Health, National Institute of Neurological Disorders and Stroke (NINDS) (1R01NS123687091).

Shahid M. Nimjee, MD, PhD
Department of Neurosurgery
The Ohio State University Wexner Medical Center
N-1014 Doan Hall
410 West 10th Avenue
Columbus, OH 43235, USA

E-mail address:
shahid.nimjee@osumc.edu

Venous Anatomy of the Central Nervous System

Maksim Shapiro, MD[a,b], Charlotte Chung, MD, PhD[a,b], Vera Sharashidze, MD[a,b], Erez Nossek, MD[a,b], Peter Kim Nelson, MD[a,b], Eytan Raz, MD, PhD[a,b,*]

KEYWORDS

- Cerebral veins • Cortical veins • Dural sinus • Labbe • Trolard • Galen • Rosenthal • Dural fistula

KEY POINTS

- Venous neuroembryology is critical in appreciating the full spectrum of venous physiology and pathophysiology, including a vast array of "normal" variants, such as developmental venous anomalies, and pathologic processes such as, for example, Vein of Galen malformations, SturgeWeber syndrome, AVM, or dural fistulas.
- The dural sinuses collect and drain most of the blood from the brain and have a predilection to form at the interface between dural folds resulting in named major dural sinuses at classical locations, but unnamed dural venous channels can exist anywhere within the dural sheaths.
- The supratentorial superficial cortical venous system is highly variable in size and arrangement with commonly seen numerous eponymic anastomotic veins of the convexity which are associated with large variability in regard to size, drainage territory, and the presence or lack of anastomotic interconnections among them.
- The deep venous system, consisting of deep medullary veins draining into the subependymal internal cerebral vein system and eventually the vein of Galen, serves the deep gray matter and deep and periventricular white matter. The deep white matter is an area of "watershed" between superficial and deep venous systems, with its own physiologic and pathologic balance.
- The spinal venous system is divided into 4 systems: the intrinsic intramedullary system; extrinsic cord surface system; extradural system; and external paravertebral system.

INTRODUCTION

Our understanding of venous anatomy of the central nervous system relies on the early work of the giants in our field including the embryologic work of Dorcas Padget,[1] and expanded by Yun Peng Huang, Raybaud, and Lasjaunias-Berenstein-Ter Brugge,[2–4] Rhoton,[5] and many others, while Armin Thron work is a key reference for spinal venous anatomy.[6] More recent perspectives are also available.[7,8] Altogether, what we know comes from a synthesis of existing anatomical works and a far less perfect understanding of functional anatomy.[9]

EMBRYOLOGY

While arterial development typically garners more attention, understanding venous neuroembryology is indispensable for comprehending the complete spectrum of venous physiology and pathophysiology, including a vast array of "normal" variants, nonpathological anatomic findings such as developmental venous anomalies, and pathologic processes including Vein of Galen aneurysms, Sturge-Weber syndrome, and dural fistulas.[7]

As the neural tube closes, reliance on simple diffusion becomes insufficient to meet the demands

[a] Department of Radiology and Neurosurgery, NYU Langone Health, New York, NY 10016, USA; [b] Department of Radiology and Neurosurgery, Bellevue Hospital Center, New York, NY 10016, USA
* Corresponding author. Department of Radiology and Neurosurgery, NYU Langone Health, 660 First Avenue, New York, NY 10016.
E-mail address: eytan.raz@gmail.com

Neurosurg Clin N Am 35 (2024) 273–286
https://doi.org/10.1016/j.nec.2024.03.001
1042-3680/24/© 2024 Elsevier Inc. All rights reserved.

of growing tissue and an arteriovenous plexus, the meninx primitiva, envelops the tube on the outside. Invagination of the same meninx into the tube gives rise to the choroid plexus. Drainage of the thin neural tissue at this stage is therefore centrifugal (inside to outside), while that of the internal choroid plexus is centripetal (outside to inside). With continued growth, coalescence of meninx primitiva into future dural sinuses and early surface venous channels takes place; some of these will regress due to continued development of the brain and skull. Maturation of transverse and sigmoid sinuses is dictated early on by development of brainstem structures, rather than the comparatively insignificant neocortex which grows subsequently.

Venous channels which form later in development (torcular and basal vein) are prone to more variations than those established early on (**Fig. 1**). Development of basal ganglia and other deep structures leads to emergence of the paired internal cerebral venous system draining in centripetal fashion toward the primitive Vein of Markowski, of which the terminal part remains as the Vein of Galen.[3]

Tremendous growth of the neopallial cortex leads to emergence of robust surface venous channels such as Rolando, Trolard, Labbe, and superficial Sylvian veins. The balance between the superficial and deep venous systems, with a "watershed" in the deep white matter, is exemplified by frequent persistence of venous arrangements favoring either superficial or deep drainage, known as developmental venous anomalies, and by extreme variants such as absence of effective superficial drainage in Sturge-Weber syndrome.[10] Venous development continues postnatally, including the maturation of connections between the Sylvian veins and cavernous sinus, and the relative diminution of the occipital sinus.

THE DURAL SINUSES

The dural sinuses play a pivotal role in draining blood from the brain, with individual dominance or prominence varying significantly due to the distribution of venous tributaries[2,9] (**Fig. 2**).[11] Predilection for major venous channels to form at the interface between dural folds results in named major dural sinuses at classical locations, namely the superior sagittal, inferior sagittal, straight, transverse, and sigmoid sinuses.[12]

Primarily draining paramedian cortical veins, meningeal veins, and veins of the falx cerebri, the superior sagittal sinus (SSS) is classically depicted as a single midline channel originating near the crista galli and terminating at the torcula, although it is often found to deviate from the midline and may be fenestrated or divided into more than 1 dural channels (see **Fig. 1**).

SSS hypoplasia (**Fig. 3**) is common in the anterior third with length of rostral sinus, as early anterior contributors are generally limited in number and size, not infrequently draining via small frontal diploic/emissary pathways. In the setting of rare SSS hypoplasia, venous drainage can be shifted to parasagittal frontal veins that drain more posteriorly in the sinus, larger diploic or emissary veins, the cavernous sinus, vein of the foramen cecum draining to paranasal mucosa and facial veins, inferior sagittal sinus, and even the deep venous system. In such cases, ligation and/or transection of the anterior third of the SSS is often safe.

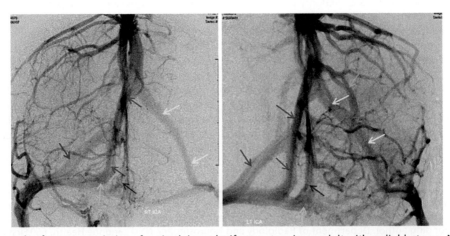

Fig. 1. Example of extreme variation of sagittal sinus plexiform nature in an adult with a glioblastoma. Notice the different venous outflow from right and left carotid injections, stressing how in order to understand the intracranial veins all the different territories should be imaged during angiography. There is splaying of the distal superior sagittal sinus in multiple limbs with multiple duplications/fenestrations. This appearance is a reminder of the plexiform nature of dural sinuses in embryos, which mostly then fuse in single channels.

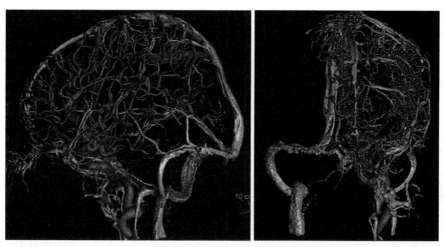

Fig. 2. Lateral and frontal projection of an arterial and venous-3D-digital subtraction angiography (DSA) (AV-3D DSA), a 3D-DSA algorithm, which allows the concurrent yet distinct display of the arterial and venous structures, which may be useful for different clinical and educational purposes.[11]

However, in a subset of patients, a dominant frontal or Sylvian vein draining into the anterior third of the superior sagittal sinus renders it functional,[13] and therefore taking the sinus would risk venous congestion and/or infarct (**Fig. 4**).

The inferior sagittal sinus extends along the free edge of the falx cerebri, draining the corpus callosum, cingulate gyrus, and medial frontal lobes, eventually joining the vein of Galen to form the straight sinus. It is highly variable in course and caliber—often diminutive—but occasionally prominent (particularly when the SSS is hypoplastic; **Fig. 5**). The straight sinus, like the SSS, can be paramedian (instead of midline) and duplicated (or even triplicated).

Classical disposition of the torcular Herophili is centrally located confluence of SSS and straight sinuses, from which bilateral transverse sinuses arise. Numerous variant configurations of the torcular exist, with common configurations including multiple channels at the confluence, early bifurcation of the superior sagittal and/or straight sinus with drainage of each limb to the ipsilateral transverse sinus, drainage of the SSS and straight sinus to 1 transverse sinus—either the same one with hypoplasia/aplasia of the contralateral transverse sinus, or each draining to separate unconnected transverse sinuses.[12]

The paired transverse sinuses receive contributions from the vein of Labbe, superior petrosal sinus, cerebellar veins, as well as diploic and occasionally extra-cranial veins. They are often asymmetric in size with the right frequently dominant, presumably due to preferential transmission of pulsation from the right atrium. Exiting the tentorium, the transverse sinus continues as the sigmoid sinus along the mastoid portion of the temporal bone and drains into the internal jugular vein at the jugular bulb, communicating with condylar veins, emissary veins, and the vertebral

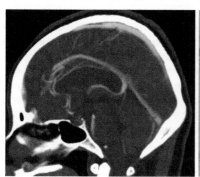
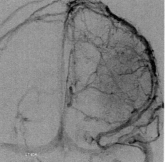
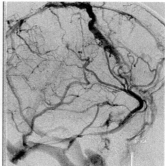

Fig. 3. Balance of venous drainage exemplified in a case of hypoplastic SSS in which something else will be larger to compensate; in this case, notice the large diploic vein, for example, taking care of the venous outflow.

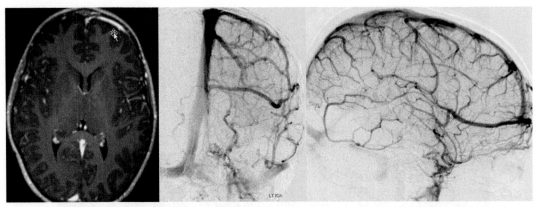

Fig. 4. Example of a dangerous variant, a functional anterior portion of superior sagittal sinus, which should be kept in mind against the general neurosurgical idea that the anterior third of the superior sagittal sinus can be safely sacrificed almost all the time. Normally, few veins drain into the anterior third of the SSS, and these usually have collaterals. However, occasionally, a large frontal or Sylvian vein happens to drain anteriorly. Taking this sinus means risking a venous infarct. Here is an extreme example of dominant inferior left frontal vein draining into the anterior third of the frontal sinus, on MRI and on angiography.

venous plexus along its course. Typically, left-right dominance of the sigmoid sinus and internal jugular vein is concordant with that of the transverse sinus; a small jugular foramen suggests developmental hypoplasia of the ipsilateral transverse-sigmoid sinus complex. Of note, there

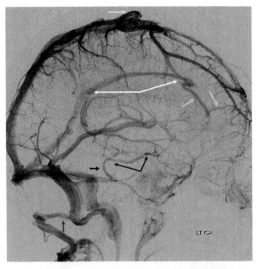

Fig. 5. Example of a very large inferior sagittal sinus (white). Why is this sinus so large? Veins are like rivers—the inferior sagittal sinus happens to be receiving a completely benign, nonpathologic mesial anterior frontal vein (light blue *arrows*). However, the increased inflow into the Galen system has likely resulted in alternate drainage of the basal vein (purple) into the superior petrosal sinus via the lateral mesencephalic vein (black)—see deep venous system and veins of posterior fossa pages for more info. Notice also a large transosseous emissary vein (pink).

are always exceptions to the rule—the sigmoid sinus can enlarge (compared to the ipsilateral transverse sinus) after receiving inflow from a prominent vein of Labbe, and mastoid emissary veins or condylar veins diverting flow from a dominant transverse-sigmoid sinus complex can result in a smaller internal jugular vein downstream—especially when the latter is compressed between the styloid process and the C1 lateral mass.

The occipital sinus, extending along the occipital bone from the torcula region to the marginal sinus of the foramen magnum or sigmoid sinus, is an embryonic sinus that infrequently persists into adulthood. When present, it varies in location and size and occasionally can be the major cerebral venous drainage pathway in the setting of absent/thrombosed transverse sinus or an arteriovenous shunting lesion, potentially complicating posterior fossa surgical approaches.

The cavernous sinuses (**Fig. 6**) are paired dural venous channels at the skull base between the Meckel's caves and sella, connected by the intercavernous (or circular) venous plexus anteriorly and posteriorly to the pituitary stalk. The cavernous sinuses are complex multicompartmental structures receiving both extracranial venous drainage (nasal, orbital, facial soft tissues) via the superior and inferior ophthalmic veins, and intracranial superficial Sylvian vein (directly or via sphenoparietal sinus), deep Sylvian vein via the basal vein of Rosenthal, and the posterior fossa via petrosal or bridging veins. Major egress includes the superior petrosal sinus to the transverse/sigmoid sinus, inferior petrosal sinus to the jugular bulb, emissary veins to the pterygoid

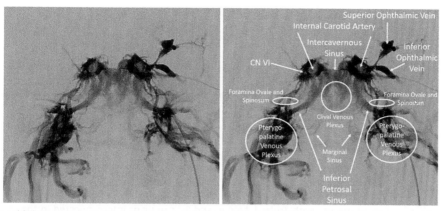

Fig. 6. Normal bilateral cavernous sinus anatomy as demonstrated with a frontal projection DSA during inferior petrosal sinus sampling, unlabeled and labeled.

venous plexus, intercavernous channels to the contralateral sinus, and clival plexus to the marginal sinus or jugular veins. Variations in cavernous sinus drainage pattern and dominance are common, and compartments within a cavernous sinus may be isolated from other portions of the same sinus (the laterocavernous sinus)[14](**Fig. 7**). Flow reversal in cavernous sinus (toward the ophthalmic veins) may be occasionally encountered in apparently normal circumstances, and often in pathologic settings such as arteriovenous shunting and increased intracranial pressure.

In addition to the major dural sinuses, unnamed dural venous channels can normally exist anywhere within the dura sheaths, and in pathologic states with increased demand for venous egress. One likely example is the persistence of the falcine sinus, an embryonic sinus located along the parietal falx, in association with vein of Galen malformation or other regional arteriovenous shunting lesions. Dural venous channels also exist as incidental variants, receiving flow from cortical/

bridging veins and draining toward 1 of the major dural sinuses. They are the rule, not exception, in the tentorium[15] and increasingly recognized in the supratentorial compartment.[16] Surgical importance of such channels lies in the risk of venous infarction from inadvertent injury during dural incision.

THE CORTICAL VEINS

The supratentorial superficial cortical venous system, predominantly draining the cortex and the subcortical white matter, is again highly variable in size and arrangement (**Figs. 8–10**). This system includes small surface veins that merge into larger cortical bridging veins, traversing the subdural space to connect with the dural sinuses. These veins can be categorized into 2 groups: a superomedial group, draining into the superior and inferior sagittal sinuses, and an inferolateral group that drains to the transverse/sigmoid and cavernous sinuses.

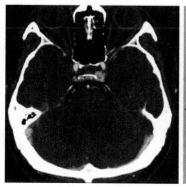
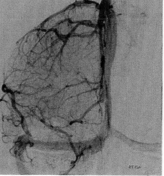
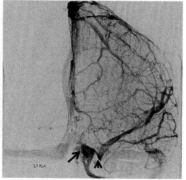

Fig. 7. Example of asymmetric cavernous sinuses as shown in a head CTA, often misdiagnosed as a carotid cavernous fistula. Angiography shows that the left cavernous sinus is larger since it receives outflow of a dominant deep middle cerebral vein, while on the right side, the dominant outflow is through a vein of Labbe.

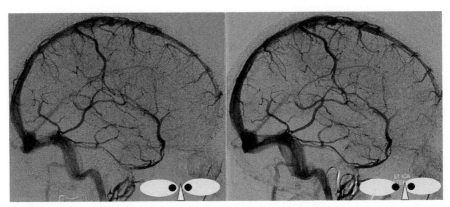

Fig. 8. Example of balanced pattern with Trolard, Labbe, and Sylvian veins interconnected in the region of the posterior Sylvian fissure.

Key anastomotic veins on the brain convexity include the superior anastomotic vein of Trolard, typically found along the parietal convexity in the postcentral sulcus and the vein of Rolando along the same sulcus (anterior to the Troland), both draining toward the superior sagittal sinus. The inferior anastomotic vein of Labbe, running laterally along the temporal convexity, typically drains posteriorly toward the transverse or sigmoid sinus. The superficial Sylvian vein (or superficial middle cerebral vein) collects blood from the opercular region and has multiple potential drainage pathways,

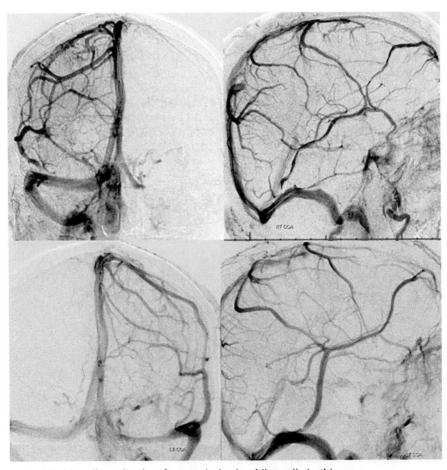

Fig. 9. Example of highly collateralized surface cortical veins, bilaterally in this case.

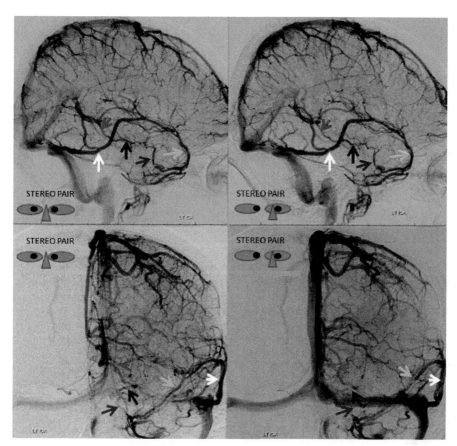

Fig. 10. Stereo pair crossed eyes showing an example of collateral connections between the Labbe (white) and Superficial Sylvian (blue) veins. Notice the fully developed basal vein of Rosenthal (posterior segment: pink; middle segment: black; anterior segment: purple), connecting the cavernous sinus to the vein of Galen and draining in both directions. Notice the superimposed deep middle cerebral vein (blue *arrow*) connected through the Sylvian vein with an anastomotic connection to the left vein of Labbe (*white arrow*).

including the sphenoparietal sinus, cavernous sinus, the pterygopalatine venous plexus, diploic/emissary veins, or via an inferior temporal vein to the superior petrosal sinus.

The balance between superficial anastomotic veins concerns their relative size (reflecting volume of drainage territory) and their extent of interconnectedness. Larger size of one or more superficial convexity veins is accompanied by correspondingly smaller size of others. The extent of connectivity between superficial veins varies widely (see **Figs. 9** and **10**). The more dominant and isolated a cortical vein is, the higher the risk of venous infarction in its territory should it become occluded by disease or surgical/endovascular compromise.

THE DEEP VENOUS SYSTEM

The deep venous system, consisting of deep medullary veins emptying into the subependymal internal cerebral vein (ICV) system and eventually the vein of Galen, drains the deep gray matter and deep/periventricular white matter (structures supplied by perforating lenticulostriate arteries). According to location in relation to the lateral ventricles, ICV tributaries can be classified into the medial group, namely septal veins, medial atrial vein, and the ICV itself, and the lateral group, including longitudinal thalamostriate/caudate veins, anterior caudate vein, lateral atrial vein, and others. Alternatively, the ICV system can be understood as an outer ring (longitudinal veins of the caudate and lateral ventricle) and an inner ring (ICV and basal veins) with multiple interconnecting veins[9] (**Fig. 11**). The classic appearance of the thalamostriate vein transitioning to the ICV at the venous angle located at the foramen of Monro is reflected by dominant outer-inner ring connection at the venous arcade at the foramen of Monro[2] (**Fig. 12**). Interruptions of the outer ring and prominence of one or more of the other interconnecting veins conceptually explain the venous

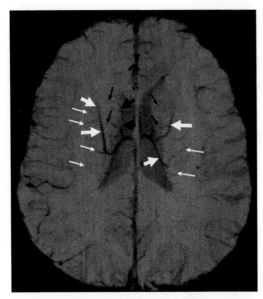

Fig. 11. SWI axial image showing the longitudinal caudate veins (thick *white arrows*), anterior caudate vein (thick *black arrows*), transverse caudate veins (thin *black arrows*), and transverse medullary deep white matter veins (thin *white arrows*).

rerouting seen in variant configurations of the ICV system (**Fig. 13**).

Within the white matter, superficial medullary veins drain the subcortical tissues centrifugally toward pial (transcortical) veins into the superficial cortical venous system, while deep medullary veins drain centripetally toward the subependymal internal cerebral venous system. Anastomotic transmedullary veins connecting the superficial and deep medullary veins allow for balance between the superficial and deep venous systems. Individual variation in the number and capacity of these anastomotic veins may contribute to variability in tolerance of outcomes (infarction or not) in the setting of deep venous occlusive or congestive states (**Fig. 14**).

The basal vein of Rosenthal, partially draining the deep white matter via the inferior ventricular vein, courses along the inferior surface of the brain, curves around the midbrain next to the anterior choroidal artery, before merging with the ICV to form the vein of Galen. It is thus strictly superficial in location, yet is often considered part of the deep venous system due to difficult surgical access and related morbidity (for example in the AVM Spetzler-Martin grading system). In its full expression, the basal vein is an unbroken conduit between the cavernous sinus and the Galen, divided in three segments. The anterior segment, from the cavernous sinus to ambient cistern, drains the anterior cerebral and deep Sylvian (middle cerebral) vein territories. The middle segment, curving over the midbrain and posterior segment extending to the vein of Galen harbor, anastomoses with ICV system, collects tributaries from the inferior temporal lobe, brainstem, and sometimes cerebellum, and connects with the lateral mesencephalic vein (which provides a potential outflow pathway). Any of these segments can be hypoplastic resulting in variations in basal vein drainage pattern (**Fig. 15**).

Developmental Venous Anomaly (DVA): Briefly, the DVA as we know it now (term coined by Lasjaunias), or medullary venous malformation as called by Yun Peng Huang,[17] is a prominent vestige of the normally inconspicuous transcerebral venous network—small veins connecting the subependymal network which drains into internal cerebral vein (or fourth ventricular veins such as the vein of the lateral recess) and the superficial venous system of the cortex or the cerebellum. These connections traverse the deep white matter and have the potential, over time, to partially compensate for constraints of either superficial or deep venous systems. Hypoplasia of some portion of the deep medullary veins could be compensated by superficial drainage of the affected territory via a transmedullary vein, resulting in a "superficial" DVA. The reverse hypoplasia of subcortical centrifugal veins with prominent

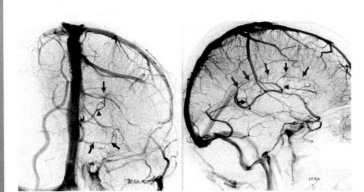

Fig. 12. Classic thalamostriate vein anatomy. Longitudinal caudate venous arcade is shown with purple arrows and within the white-bordered regions below. Classic Monro opening with arrowhead. Inferior ventricular vein collects the posterior portion of the arcade and is shown in black arrows.

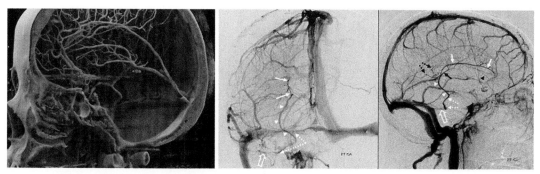

Fig. 13. Cinematic rendering of dynaCT, frontal and lateral angiography, showing caudate veins (*white arrows*) drain via the inferior ventricular vein (white *arrowheads*) into the lateral mesencephalic vein (dashed *white arrows*) and then into the superior petrosal sinus (open *white arrow*). (*Courtesy of* Matthew Young, DO).

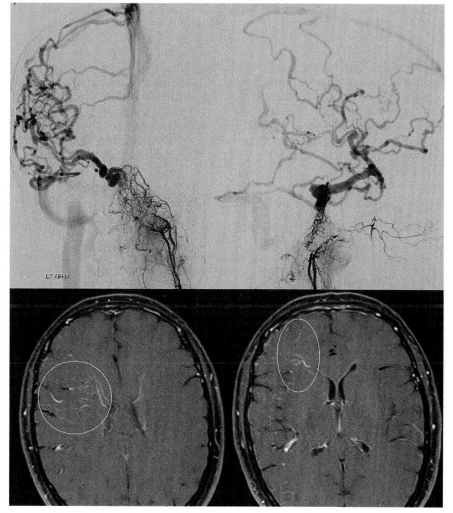

Fig. 14. Cavernous sinus dural arteriovenous fistula with supply from the ascending pharyngeal and drainage intracranial via the Sylvian veins. Notice prominence of transmedullary veins in the right centrum semiovale on post contrast T1. The transmedullary veins, connecting the superficial and deep medullary veins allow for balance between the superficial and deep venous systems, contributing to tolerance in congestive states.

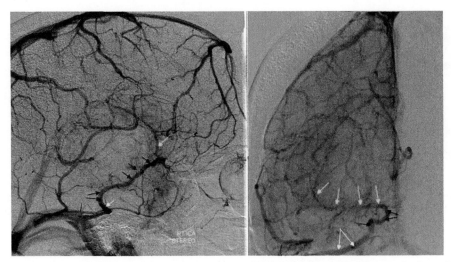

Fig. 15. Example of anterior (telencephalic and diencephalic) basal vein (blue) draining via the lateral mesencephalic vein (purple) into the superior petrosal sinus (yellow). This is an example in which the posterior 2 segments of the basal vein of Rosenthal are atretic with variant drainage of the anterior segment.

deep drainage of the area is a deep-draining DVA. The "Developmental Venous Anomaly" term emphasizes its developmental nature, and Medullary Venous Malformation name is more reflective of the white matter, medullary location of the vein, and its essentially non-pathologic nature other than rare exceptions.[18]

The transmedullar venous system plays a major role in compensation—either from occlusive states (venous thrombosis) or congestion (dural fistula and others). For example, when the Galen is overwhelmed congested by a shunt such as the falcotentorial dural fistula, the trans-cerebral network can help drain the internal cerebral vein, averting disaster. Alternatively, when the superficial system is dysfunctional, for example, in cases of Sturge-Weber syndrome, the trans-cerebral network of medullary veins is prominent in compensation. However, in most instances, such life-saving measures are not necessary.

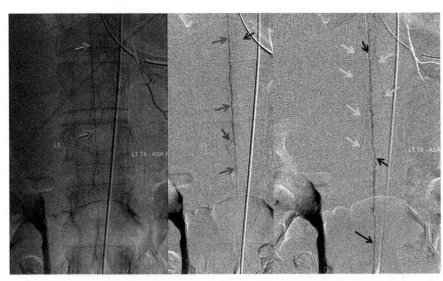

Fig. 16. Example of veins as seen from Adamkiewicz (red) injection. You can faintly see tiny dots to the left of the anterior spinal artery in the middle image—those are sulco-comissural arteries, seen end-on. In the venous phase, notice a single (usually dorsal) longitudinal vein (dark blue) and multiple radicular veins (light blue) on surfaces of the cauda roots.

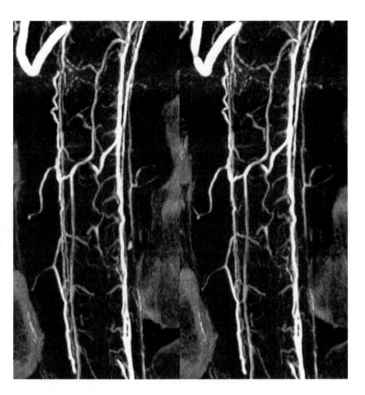

Fig. 17. Cervical spinal cord stereo maximum intensity projection (MIPs) showing dorsal and ventral-draining veins.

VENOUS ANATOMY OF THE SPINE

The venous system is, in many ways, more important in understanding pathophysiology of spinal vascular disease than the arterial one. Far more important than the arterial counterparts[19–21] are the varied and imperfectly understood injuries to the cord inflicted by dysfunction of the venous apparatus—venous hypertension, high-flow venopathy, and outflow obstruction.[22,23] The prototypical vascular condition of the cord—dural AV fistula—manifests its clinical and anatomic consequences as progressive venous failure.

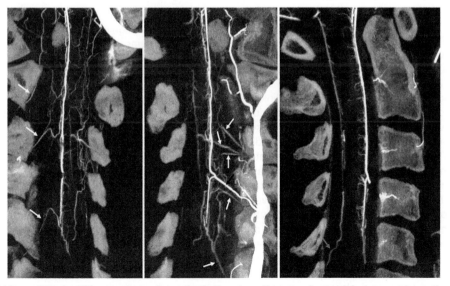

Fig. 18. Oblique MIPs in different planes from CBCT, showing all types of veins. Black arrow is on the radiculo-medullary artery. There is a lot of variability in the extent of normal radicular venous drainage, which for example, plays a role in symptomatology of spinal dural fistulas.

Broadly speaking, the spinal venous system can be divided into 4 systems/components, with the functional barrier between these systems being the dura.[6]

1. Intrinsic (intramedullary/intrinsic cord veins)
2. Extrinsic (cord surface veins and the radicular/ bridging veins which allow venous outflow to traverse the dura)
3. Extradural (epidural plexi and drainage into the bony spinal canal outside dura)
4. External (osseous, paravertebral, etc—anything outside the epidural space).

The intradural (intrinsic and extrinsic cord) and extradural (epidural plexus, paravertebral) systems are highly redundant and therefore fail only under extreme circumstances. The weak links, and therefore site of pathology, are the transdural connections—radiculomedullary and bridging veins. These veins are relatively limited, and have no effective alternative pathway for venous egress through the dural cover. Their paucity and failure is as much responsible for symptoms of dural arteriovenous fistula as the shunt-related pathologic inflow.

The visualization of spinal veins is challenging. For the intrinsic system, the commercially available noninvasive imaging has essentially no role since the intrinsic cord veins are below MRI resolution. Cone beam computed tomography (CBCT) and 2D-digital subtraction angiography (DSA) are probably the best complementary methods of acquiring spatial and temporal venous information.[22,24]

Regarding the extrinsic system, cord surface veins are inconsistently seen on MRI, but they are well seen when injecting the dominant artery (Adamkiewicz) by DSA and CBCT (**Fig. 16**). Bridging and radicular veins can be seen surprisingly well on high-res T2. They are well seen on CBCT and DSA if a large enough spinal artery is injected (**Figs. 17–19**).

The radicular and bridging veins are the link between the intradural (cord) and extradural (epidural) venous systems and it is the weakest point in the whole system. They are limited in number. Their paucity determines the extent of clinical symptomatology in spinal dural fistulas— and it is important to visualize and understand them. On the one hand, there are "radicular" veins which follow the nerve roots (dorsal and ventral) into the nerve root sleeve, through the dura, and into the foraminal or epidural venous systems. The "bridging" veins also connect the surface cord veins with extradural venous systems, but not exiting via nerve root sleeve or, in a broad sense, somehow not connected to the radicular nerves. The less radicular/bridging veins one

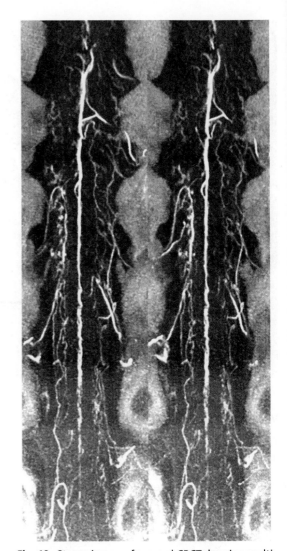

Fig. 19. Stereo image of coronal CBCT showing multiple radicular veins in a normal subject, following injection of the supreme intercostal artery.

has, the more the chance that a fistula or something else congesting the cord may not be as well tolerated.

For the extrinsic venous network, paravertebral and epidural plexi, normal arterial injections are generally not good for visualizing this venous system—too many arterial tributaries, and only one can be injected at a time. Pathology (IVC thrombosis, fistulas) congest these plexuses, making them visible, but such conditions are not representative of the normal venous architecture (**Fig. 20**). The rich network of veins all around the vertebral column and ventral and dorsal epidural venous plexi constitute a highly capacious and quite effective drainage system which parallels that of the inferior vena cava. This system is nowadays

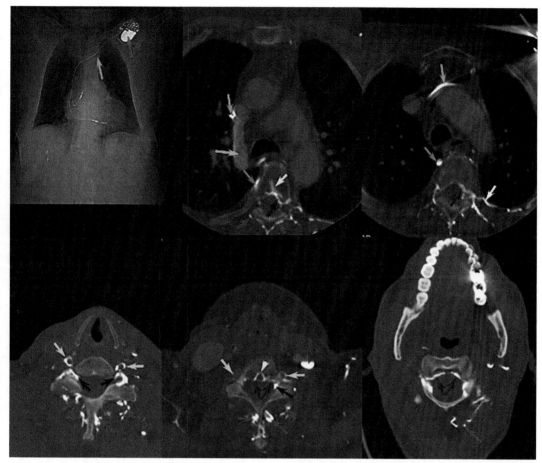

Fig. 20. Example of reflux of intravenous contrast administered into an upper extremity in an individual with distal venous outflow obstruction (orange *arrows*) (from pacemaker) as a way to visualize the extrinsic spinal venous network. Notice the anterior epidural plexus (purple) and the medullary veins draining into a venous network within and around the nerve sheath (dark blue) which is named "emissary veins." An extensive paraspinal network subserving the posterior elements and adjacent musculature is present (pink). The longitudinal efferents eventually drain into the azygos system (light green).

maximally understood and images during spinal venous angiography performed for treatment of CSF venous fistulas.

SUMMARY

To understand the veins of the central venous system, a functional non-compartmentalized perspective of the system is necessary, appreciating the overall balance between various classically separate components of the global system, paired by appropriate utilization of cross-sectional imaging tools and attentive angiography.

DISCLOSURE

Dr.E.Raz is a Consultant at Balt, Cerenovus, Imperative Care, Medtronic, Phenox, Qapel, Vasorum, and a Proctor at Microvention.

REFERENCES

1. Padget DH. The cranial venous system in man in reference to development, adult configuration, and relation to the arteries. Am J Anat 1956;98(3):307–55.
2. Salamon G, Huang Yun P, Michotey P, et al. Radiologic anatomy of the brain. Berlin, Heidelberg: Springer; 1976.
3. Charles R. Normal and abnormal embryology and development of the intracranial vascular system. Neurosurg Clin 2010;21(3):399–426.
4. Lasjaunias P, Berenstein A, Brugge Karel G. Clinical vascular anatomy and variations. Berlin, Heidelberg: Springer Berlin Heidelberg; 2001.
5. Rhoton Jr, Albert L. Rhoton's cranial anatomy and surgical approaches. Oxford University Press; 2019.
6. Thron Armin K. Vascular anatomy of the spinal cord: neuroradiologic investigations and clinical syndromes. New York: Springer; 1988.

7. Shapiro M, Raz E, Nossek E, et al. Cerebral venous anatomy: implications for the neurointerventionalist. J NeuroIntervent Surg 2022. https://doi.org/10.1136/neurintsurg-2022-018917. neurintsurg-2022-018917.

8. Ota T. Functional Cerebral Venous Anatomy from the Viewpoint of Venous Collaterals Part I, Supratentorial Superficial and Deep Venous System. SVIN 2023; e001050. https://doi.org/10.1161/SVIN.123.001050.

9. Lasjaunias P, Berenstein A, Brugge Karel G. Intracranial venous system. In: Lasjaunias P, Berenstein A, Brugge Karel G, editors. Clinical vascular anatomy and variations. Berlin, Heidelberg: Springer; 2001. p. 631–713.

10. Bentson JR, Wilson GH, Newton TH. Cerebral venous drainage pattern of the Sturge-Weber syndrome. Radiology 1971;101(1):111–8.

11. Raz E, Shapiro M, Mir O, et al. Arterial and venous 3D fusion AV-3D-DSA: a novel approach to cerebrovascular neuroimaging. Am J Neuroradiol 2021; 42(7):1282–4.

12. Joseph Shamfa C, Elias R, Tubbs R. Variations of the intracranial dural venous sinuses. Anatomy, imaging and surgery of the intracranial dural venous sinuses. Elsevier; 2020. p. 205–20.

13. Sahoo Sushanta K, Ghuman Mandeep S, Salunke Pravin, et al. Evaluation of anterior third of superior sagittal sinus in normal population: identifying the subgroup with dominant drainage. J Neurosci Rural Pract 2016;7(2):257–61.

14. Gailloud P, San Millán Ruíz D, Muster M, et al. Angiographic anatomy of the laterocavernous sinus. AJNR Am J Neuroradiol 2000;21(10):1923–9.

15. Matsushima T, Suzuki SO, Fukui M, et al. Microsurgical anatomy of the tentorial sinuses. J Neurosurg 1989;71(6):923–8.

16. Shapiro M, Srivatanakul K, Raz E, et al. Dural venous channels: hidden in plain sight–reassessment of an under-recognized entity. AJNR Am J Neuroradiol 2020;41(8):1434–40.

17. Okudera T, Huang YP, Fukusumi A, et al. Micro-angiographical studies of the medullary venous system of the cerebral hemisphere. Neuropathology 1999;19(1):93–111.

18. Pereira Vitor M, Geibprasert S, Krings T, et al. Pathomechanisms of symptomatic developmental venous anomalies. Stroke 2008;39(12):3201–15.

19. Haynes J, Shapiro M, Raz E, et al. Intra-arterial thrombolytic therapy for acute anterior spinal artery stroke. J Clin Neurosci 2021;84:102–5.

20. Renieri L, Raz E, Lanzino G, et al. Spinal artery aneurysms: clinical presentation, radiological findings and outcome. J Neurointerv Surg 2018;10(7):644–8.

21. Shlobin Nathan A, Raz E, Shapiro M, et al. Spinal neurovascular complications with anterior thoracolumbar spine surgery: a systematic review and review of thoracolumbar vascular anatomy. Neurosurg Focus 2020;49(3):E9.

22. Shapiro M, Nossek E, Vera S, et al. Spinal dural and epidural fistulas: role of cone beam CT in diagnosis and treatment. J NeuroIntervent Surg 2023. https://doi.org/10.1136/jnis-2022-019950. jnis-2022-019950.

23. Shapiro M, Kister I, Raz E, et al. Spinal dural fistula and anterior spinal artery supply from the same segmental artery: Case report of volumetric T2 MRI diagnosis and rational endovascular treatment. Interv Neuroradiol 2019;25(5):579–84.

24. Raz E, Nossek E, Sahlein Daniel H, et al. Principles, techniques and applications of high resolution cone beam CT angiography in the neuroangio suite. J Neurointerventional Surg 2022. https://doi.org/10.1136/jnis-2022-018722.

Idiopathic Intracranial Hypertension

Matthew Anderson, MD[a], Eliza Baird-Daniel, MD[a], Raymond Michael Meyer, MD[a], Michael R. Levitt, MD[a,b,c,d,e],*

KEYWORDS

- Idiopathic intracranial hypertension • Venous sinus stent • Pseudotumor cerebri

KEY POINTS

- Patients with symptoms of idiopathic intracranial hypertension should be assessed for underlying intracranial venous hypertension and/or dural venous sinus stenosis.
- Dural venous stenting can be considered a first-line treatment for patients with idiopathic intracranial hypertension who meet diagnostic criteria and dural venous sinus pressure gradient thresholds associated with an area of stenosis.
- A diagnostic framework that separates patients with and without intracranial venous stenosis can be used to direct treatment in patients with idiopathic intracranial hypertension.

INTRODUCTION/HISTORY

Idiopathic Intracranial hypertension (IIH), also called pseudotumor cerebri, is a disease most commonly found in overweight women of child-bearing age.[1] It is characterized by migrainous headaches and progressive visual loss. IIH was originally described as "meningitis serosa," attributed to an increase in cerebrospinal fluid (CSF) secretion due to dysfunction of the autonomic nervous system.[2] An alternative hypothesis was middle ear disease leading to aseptic meningitis and subsequent hyperproduction of CSF resulting in an increase in intracranial pressure (ICP).[2] This led to it being renamed "otitic hydrocephalus." In the 1930s, ventriculography studies demonstrated that ventricular size did not change in IIH patients, which led investigators to debate the mechanism that caused increased ICP despite a lack of radiographic correlation on ventriculography.[2] The condition was renamed "pseudotumor cerebri" given its clinical features of increased ICP typically observed in patients with intracranial neoplasms.[3]

In 1955, Foley[4] authored a paper abandoning the term pseudotumor cerebri and instead terming it as benign intracranial hypertension, due to the normal CSF composition and lack of ventriculomegaly. Subsequently, ophthalmology societies shifted the nomenclature from benign intracranial hypertension to IIH, since the "benign" terminology did not account for the debilitating visual loss caused by the disease.[5]

The pathophysiologic explanation of IIH previously focused on increased CSF production. Original treatments focused on decreasing CSF production through medications (such as acetazolamide) or CSF diversion via ventriculoperitoneal or lumboperitoneal shunting. Recently, abnormally high dural venous sinus pressure, whether due to focal venous sinus stenosis (seen in the majority of IIH patients) or globally elevated central venous pressure, has been identified as a key pathophysiological driver of IIH. Since absorption of CSF into the dural venous sinuses requires a pressure differential (typically 3–5 mm Hg) across the arachnoid granulations, elevated dural

[a] Department of Neurological Surgery, University of Washington, Seattle, WA, USA; [b] Stroke & Applied Neuroscience Center, University of Washington, Seattle, WA, USA; [c] Department of Radiology, University of Washington, Seattle, WA, USA; [d] Department of Mechanical Engineering, University of Washington, Seattle, WA, USA; [e] Department of Neurology, University of Washington, Seattle, WA, USA
* Corresponding author. 325 9th Avenue, Box 359924, Seattle, WA 98104.
E-mail address: mlevitt@uw.edu

Neurosurg Clin N Am 35 (2024) 287–291
https://doi.org/10.1016/j.nec.2024.02.001

venous sinus pressure causes venous congestion and reduces CSF absorption, increasing ICP.[6]

While it is unknown whether venous sinus stenosis is a primary cause or a result of the disease, some hypothesize that as ICP increases, extrinsic compression of the venous sinuses may worsen, contributing to further venous congestion, creating a positive feedback loop.[7] Another theory proposes that the anatomic features of the lateral transverse sinus at its junction with the sigmoid are more susceptible to extramural compression and stenosis.[6] Thus, even though there is global extramural pressure on the entire dural venous sinus system, there is added venous congestion at the transverse sinus resulting in worsening of disease presentation.[6] The goal of this article is to define the presentation, diagnostic tools, and treatment strategies for IIH with particular focus on the venous contributions of, and treatments for, the disease.

DEFINITION

IIH is defined as elevated ICP (>25 cm H_2O) without another identifiable cause.[8] One set of criteria accepts a lower diagnostic ICP threshold of 20 to 25 cm H_2O when there is presence of 1 or more of the following ancillary symptoms: pulse-synchronous tinnitus, abducens palsy, Frisen grade 2+ papilledema, absence of optic disc drusen on ultrasonography, transverse sinus stenosis, partially empty sella, or enlarged optic nerve sheaths on neuroimaging.[9] The modified Dandy criteria (**Box 1**) is the most recent classification system for IIH.[9]

The visual loss seen in IIH presents initially as transient visual obscurations and loss in visual fields.[10] Transient visual obscurations are defined as loss or clouding of vision in 1 or both eyes lasting for less than a minute, caused by transient ischemia in the optic nerve head as a result of increased ICP.[10] Initially, the visual loss that characterizes IIH is an enlarged blind spot, such as inferior partial arcuate or nasal defects.[10] As the disease becomes more severe, there is loss of visual acuity. Optical coherence tomography can be used to quantify the papilledema grade and determine structural changes to the optic nerve seen in IIH.[1]

Recently, an alternative nomenclature and classification for IIH called "chronic intracranial venous hypertension syndrome" has been proposed.[6] This stratifies patients into 4 different types based on venous pathology: craniocervical, central, mixed, and post-venous thrombosis. In the craniocervical subtype, there is elevated ICP secondary to venous sinus stenosis. In the central subtype, there is elevated ICP secondary to globally elevated central venous pressures without dural venous sinus stenosis. In the mixed subtype, there is elevated ICP secondary to both elevated central venous pressure and focal venous sinus stenosis. In the post-venous thrombosis subtype, there is elevated ICP due to ongoing or resolved dural venous sinus thrombosis. Because each subtype is defined by its venous pathophysiology, treatment options are linked to each subtype: craniocervical patients benefit from venous sinus stenting, central patients benefit from weight loss and medical therapies, while mixed type and post-venous thrombosis patients may require a combination of treatments.

TREATMENT

The goal of IIH treatment is primarily that of vision preservation, with ancillary symptoms such as headaches considered secondary concerns. Surgical treatment of IIH solely for headaches is not recommended, given the relatively high complication rates, as well as concomitant headache disorders in the IIH patient population. Thus, it is important to carefully measure patients' severity of ophthalmology symptoms prior to making any treatment decisions. A multidisciplinary team including neurosurgeons, neurointerventionalists, ophthalmologists, and headache specialists is critical to appropriate and responsible IIH treatment.

When defining a treatment plan, patients are often categorized based on the rapidity of the vision loss component of their disease. In patients with chronic IIH, vision loss is slow to progress. In patients with fulminant subtype, vision loss is rapid and severe (usually within 4 weeks of symptoms

---

Box 1
Modified Dandy criteria

- Signs and symptoms of ICP
- Absence of localizing findings on neurologic examination
- Absence of deformity, displacement, or obstruction of the ventricular system and otherwise normal neurodiagnostic studies, except for evidence of increased CSF pressure (>20 cm H_2O). Abnormal neuroimaging except for empty sella turcica, optic nerve sheath with enlarged CSF spaces and smooth-walled non–flow-related venous sinus stenosis or collapse should lead to another diagnosis
- Awake and alert
- No other cause of increased ICP

Adapted from Ref.[9]

onset and progressive over a matter of days).[8] Treatment for IIH patients thus differs based on the acuity of the disease as discussed in the following paragraphs.

The mainstay of chronic IIH treatment is weight loss, oral carbonic anhydrase inhibitors (such as acetazolamide), and, if necessary, surgical treatment. The Idiopathic Intracranial Hypertension Treatment Trial showed that maximally tolerated doses of acetazolamide in conjunction with a low-salt weight loss program led to a decrease in papilledema in IIH patients.[9] Patients with mild papilledema (Frisen grade 1–3) fared much better than those with higher grade papilledema (grade 4–5), limiting the generalizability of the study's findings in high-grade patients. In addition, while acetazolamide is generally well tolerated, some patients may develop side effects such as nausea, vomiting, dysgeusia, diarrhea, paresthesia, and fatigue, which can lead to noncompliance.[9] Pairing acetazolamide with other medications can reduce the required acetazolamide dose, which may be better tolerated. Topiramate, which has mild carbonic anhydrase inhibition and appetite suppressant, is one such option.[1] Octreotide is another medication that has been shown to decrease papilledema in patients with IIH as an adjunct to acetazolamide.[10]

Patients with progressive vision loss despite weight loss and carbonic anhydrase inhibitors, those unable to tolerate medication side effects, or those with fulminant IIH should be considered for surgical treatment. This includes CSF diversion (ventriculoperitoneal or lumboperitoneal shunt placement), optic nerve sheath fenestration, or dural venous sinus stenting. Optic nerve sheath fenestration tends to be best considered for chronic IIH patients whose main symptoms are related to vision loss, but nearly half of patients will have persistent visual symptoms after treatment, and other IIH symptoms such as headaches are not addressed with this procedure.[11] Thus, most patients who fail medical management are referred for CSF diversion surgery. A recent meta-analysis of CSF diversion for IIH found high re-treatment and complications rates, suggesting room for improvement.[12]

The contribution of dural venous sinus disease to the pathophysiology of IIH has led to the advent of endovascular venous sinus stenting as an alternative for the surgical management of patients with IIH. When compared to CSF diversion procedures, venous sinus stenting has a more favorable treatment profile. CSF diversion procedures are associated with a 7.6% major complication risk and 39.2% minor complication risk, and reoperation rates of 38% to 86% usually due to shunt infection or malfunction.[13] Venous sinus stenting series suggest a lower reoperation rate of 6% to 26%, most of which are often due to recurrent stenosis.[14,15] While CSF diversion procedures only show a 70% improvement in papilledema, venous stenting has been shown to improve papilledema in as many as 94% of patients, improve tinnitus in as many as 93% of patients, and improve visual changes in as many as 87% of patients.[13]

To evaluate for the eligibility of stenting for IIH, patients should undergo cerebral venous sinus manometry, either as a standalone diagnostic procedure or immediately prior to stent placement. This procedure involves placement of a microcatheter within the dural venous sinuses for direct transduction of cerebral venous pressures throughout the dural venous sinus system, as well as catheter venography to define any areas of venous sinus stenosis. This is best performed under minimal sedation, as general anesthesia has been found to have a variable effect on measured pressures.[16] A pressure gradient of $\geq$ 8 mm Hg between 2 sinus segments (most typically between the transverse and sigmoid sinuses), as well as normal pressure (<25 mm Hg) proximal to the sinus, is used to select patients for stent eligibility, although some studies suggest patients with pressure gradients as low as 4 mm Hg may benefit.[17] Approximately 40% of IIH patients are eligible for stent treatment using the pressure gradient threshold of $\geq$ 8 mm Hg.[18]

In IIH patients with venous sinus stenosis meeting the aforementioned criteria, stent treatment can occur either at the time of manometry or in a delayed fashion, depending on clinical circumstances. The optimal antiplatelet medication for dural venous sinus stenting has not been established, but is most commonly daily aspirin (325 mg) and clopidogrel (75 mg), which is continued for 3 to 6 months after the procedure. Point-of-care platelet function testing such as VerifyNow can be used to ensure adequate platelet inhibition. Stent placement occurs with the patient under general anesthesia, via transfemoral, transbrachial, or transjugular venous access. The patient is fully heparinized and an 8-French catheter is navigated over a 4-French, 5-French, or 6-French intermediate catheter to reach the proximal sigmoid sinus. This position is necessary to deliver the relatively stiff stents used in the dural venous sinuses.

Stent selection varies widely, and while dural venous sinus–specific stents are under development, at the time of this writing no stent is Food and Drug Administration approved for dural venous sinus stenting. Most commonly, an open-cell stent such as the Zilver (Cook Medical) is deployed across the stenosis. The diameter of the stent is often sized as close to the sinus as possible, as oversizing has been associated with the development of additional symptoms and eventual stent-adjacent stenosis.[19] If possible, telescoping stents across the entire length of the transverse sinus (from the proximal torcula through the distal sigmoid sinus) may be advisable to avoid stent-adjacent stenosis. When bilateral stenosis is present, the more dominant sinus or the sinus with the greater amount of stenosis is chosen as the sole sinus for stenting; simultaneous bilateral stenting is not required.

Postoperatively, patients can be observed overnight in the ward, or discharged home on the same day as the stent procedure.[20] Perioperative complications are seen in up to 7.4% after venous sinus stenting and include subdural hematoma, cerebellar hemorrhage, and stent-associated stenosis.[5] The most common reported complication was new ipsilateral headache (reported in 20%–100%), though this often resolves in a few days. More serious complications include intracranial hemorrhage (4%–6%) and stent-adjacent stenosis.[21]

A proposed treatment algorithm has been developed for IIH patients based on the aforementioned. For those with fulminant disease without venous sinus stenosis, CSF diversion should be considered first-line therapy as these patients are at greatest risk of loss of visual acuity. In patients with venous sinus stenosis and fulminant disease, urgent venous sinus manometry should be considered to determine stent eligibility, and stent placement should occur as soon as possible if patients meet manometry criteria; otherwise, CSF diversion surgery should take place. Fulminant IIH cases can also be temporarily treated with lumbar puncture and/or lumbar drainage.

Those with chronic IIH without venous sinus stenosis should be considered for initial conservative management with acetazolamide and weight loss, and stepwise escalation of treatment as discussed earlier. If medical management fails (due to progression of visual symptoms despite medical management, or side effect intolerance), CSF diversion surgery should be considered. Note that in all cases, venous manometry may also be performed in patients without obvious cross-sectional imaging evidence of venous sinus stenosis, since a venous pressure gradient may be seen in patients with anatomic stenosis as low as 30%.[7]

SUMMARY

The pathophysiology of IIH is multifactorial, and in many cases, cerebral venous hypertension is a contributing factor. Prompt treatment of IIH is important to protect vision and improve quality of life. Based on the acuity and severity of symptoms, medical or surgical management may be indicated. In patients meeting criteria for surgical management, and with a venous sinus pressure gradient on venous manometry, venous sinus stenting can be considered as a first-line surgical treatment for IIH.

CLINICS CARE POINTS

- Cerebral venous hypertension must be considered when evaluating a patient with IIH.
- The presence of dural venous sinus stenosis or other evidence for cerebral venous hypertension on magnetic resonance venography warrants angiographic evaluation to determine pressure gradient.
- Venous stenting is a safe intervention for patients with IIH in the setting of cerebral venous stenosis with improvement of tinnitus, vision changes, and headaches with rates comparable to that found in CSF diversion.

DISCLOSURE

M.R. Levitt received unrestricted educational grants from Stryker, United States and Medtronic, has equity interest in Synchron, Proprio, Apertur, Stroke Diagnostics, Hyperion Surgical, Stereotaxis, and Fluid Biomed, serves on the editorial board of Journal of NeuroInterventional Surgery and Frontiers in Surgery, serves on the data safety monitoring board for Arsenal Medical, and is a consultant for Aeaean Advisers and Metis Innovative. M. Anderson received unrestricted educational grants from Cerenovus and Microvention. E. Baird-Daniel and R.M. Meyer have no disclosures.

REFERENCES

1. Wang MTM, Bhatti MT, Danesh-Meyer HV. Idiopathic intracranial hypertension: Pathophysiology, diagnosis and management. J Clin Neurosci 2022;95:172–9.
2. Johnston I. The historical development of the pseudotumor concept. Neurosurg Focus 2001;11(2):E2.
3. Davidoff LM. Pseudotumor cerebri; benign intracranial hypertension. Neurology 1956;6(9):605–15.
4. Foley J. Benign forms of intracranial hypertension - "toxic" and "otitic" hydrocephalus. Brain 1955;78(1):1–41.

5. Thanki S, Guerrero W, Mokin M. Treatment of Pseudotumor Cerebri (Sinus Stenosis). Neurosurg Clin N Am 2022;33(2):207–14.

6. Fargen KM, Coffman S, Torosian T, et al. "Idiopathic" intracranial hypertension: An update from neurointerventional research for clinicians. Cephalalgia Int J Headache 2023;43(4). https://doi.org/10.1177/03331024231161323. 3331024231161323.

7. Fargen KM. Idiopathic intracranial hypertension is not idiopathic: proposal for a new nomenclature and patient classification. J Neurointerv Surg 2020; 12(2):110–4.

8. Bouffard MA. Fulminant Idiopathic Intracranial Hypertension. Curr Neurol Neurosci Rep 2020;20(4):8.

9. Wall M. Update on Idiopathic Intracranial Hypertension. Neurol Clin 2017;35(1):45–57.

10. Raoof N, Hoffmann J. Diagnosis and treatment of idiopathic intracranial hypertension. Cephalalgia Int J Headache 2021;41(4):472–8.

11. Spitze A, Malik A, Al-Zubidi N, et al. Optic nerve sheath fenestration vs cerebrospinal diversion procedures: what is the preferred surgical procedure for the treatment of idiopathic intracranial hypertension failing maximum medical therapy? J Neuro-Ophthalmol 2013;33(2):183–8.

12. Salih M, Enriquez-Marulanda A, Khorasanizadeh M, et al. Cerebrospinal Fluid Shunting for Idiopathic Intracranial Hypertension: A Systematic Review, Meta-Analysis, and Implications for a Modern Management Protocol. Neurosurgery 2022;91(4):529–40.

13. Nicholson P, Brinjikji W, Radovanovic I, et al. Venous sinus stenting for idiopathic intracranial hypertension: a systematic review and meta-analysis. J Neurointerv Surg 2019;11(4):380–5.

14. Garner RM, Aldridge JB, Wolfe SQ, et al. Quality of life, need for retreatment, and the re-equilibration phenomenon after venous sinus stenting for idiopathic intracranial hypertension. J Neurointerv Surg 2021;13(1):79–85.

15. El Mekabaty A, Obuchowski NA, Luciano MG, et al. Predictors for venous sinus stent retreatment in patients with idiopathic intracranial hypertension. J Neurointerv Surg 2017;9(12):1228–32.

16. Fargen KM, Spiotta AM, Hyer M, et al. Comparison of venous sinus manometry gradients obtained while awake and under general anesthesia before venous sinus stenting. J Neurointerv Surg 2017;9(10):990–3.

17. Inam ME, Martinez-Gutierrez JC, Kole MJ, et al. Venous Sinus Stenting for Low Pressure Gradient Stenoses in Idiopathic Intracranial Hypertension. Neurosurgery 2022;91(5):734–40.

18. Levitt MR, Hlubek RJ, Moon K, et al. Incidence and predictors of dural venous sinus pressure gradient in idiopathic intracranial hypertension and non-idiopathic intracranial hypertension headache patients: results from 164 cerebral venograms. J Neurosurg 2017;126(2):347–53.

19. Boddu SR, Gobin P, Oliveira C, et al. Anatomic measurements of cerebral venous sinuses in idiopathic intracranial hypertension patients. PLoS One 2018; 13(6):e0196275.

20. Iyer AM, Midtlien JP, Kittel C, et al. Intensive care unit admission is not necessary after venous sinus stenting. J Neurointerv Surg 2023. https://doi.org/10.1136/jnis-2023-020240. jnis-2023-020240.

21. Al-Mufti F, Dodson V, Amuluru K, et al. Neuroendovascular Cerebral Sinus Stenting in Idiopathic Intracranial Hypertension. Interv Neurol 2020;8(2–6):164–71.

Causes of Pulsatile Tinnitus and Treatment Options

Badih J. Daou, MD, Andrew F. Ducruet, MD*

KEYWORDS

- Emissary vein anomalies • Endovascular • Jugular vein anomalies • Pulsatile tinnitus • Venous
- Venous sinus stenosis • Sigmoid sinus abnormalities • Stenting

KEY POINTS

- Pulsatile tinnitus requires detailed workup. Careful evaluation of the venous sinuses, jugular bulb, and emissary veins on cerebral angiography or noninvasive vascular imaging may identify a causative venous abnormality.
- Venous causes of pulsatile tinnitus are among the most common structural pathologies and may warrant intervention.
- Endovascular treatment has demonstrated high efficacy and safety in the management of venous causes of pulsatile tinnitus.

INTRODUCTION

Tinnitus, which affects more than 740 million adults globally, can be either pulsatile or nonpulsatile.[1] Pulsatile tinnitus (PT) is defined as a rhythmic sound or noise perceived as coming from the ear and can be a debilitating symptom with significant physical and psychosocial impacts.[2] PT should be differentiated from nonpulsatile tinnitus because the 2 entities are usually related to different pathophysiological processes, and PT is much more likely to be associated with an underlying structural cause. Although PT is most often related to a benign process, it may be associated with lesions that can result in intraparenchymal hemorrhage, increased intracranial pressure, visual decline, or stroke. A thorough evaluation of the patient is essential not only for symptomatic relief but also to mitigate further neurologic consequences.

Cerebrovascular abnormalities have been implicated in the development of PT through either abnormalities of the venous system or the arterial system.[3] Advances in imaging techniques and endovascular tools have allowed an increasing number of etiologies and therapeutic options for PT to be identified.

DISCUSSION
Examination

PT can be objective or subjective. Although subjective PT is only heard by the patient, objective PT can be auscultated by the examiner with the use of a stethoscope. A bruit can sometimes be appreciated over the patient's neck, orbits, or head.[2] Compression of the jugular vein in the neck and the performance of a Valsalva maneuver are additional useful diagnostic tools. If jugular venous compression or a Valsalva maneuver improves PT, a venous cause should be suspected. However, if these maneuvers make the tinnitus louder, then an arterial cause is more likely.[4] Compression of the contralateral jugular vein may increase the intensity of PT, given increased venous outflow on the affected side. Furthermore, PT can be pulse-synchronous or asynchronous.

Department of Neurosurgery, Barrow Neurological Institute, St. Joseph's Hospital and Medical Center, Phoenix, AZ, USA

* Corresponding author. c/o Neuroscience Publications, Barrow Neurological Institute, St. Joseph's Hospital and Medical Center, 350 W Thomas Road, Phoenix, AZ 85013.
E-mail address: Neuropub@barrowneuro.org

Neurosurg Clin N Am 35 (2024) 293–303
https://doi.org/10.1016/j.nec.2024.03.002
1042-3680/24/

Pulse-synchronous PT, in synchrony with the patient's heartbeat, is more likely to be related to an underlying vascular cause, often from abnormal or turbulent blood flow within the venous sinuses. However, pulse-asynchronous PT is more likely to be related to an underlying mechanical issue that causes impaired sound conduction.[2,5]

PT is typically unilateral. A low-pitch PT tends to be venous whereas a high-pitch PT may reflect an arterial pathology or a dural arteriovenous fistula (dAVF).[2] Arterial PT tends to be louder and more bothersome to patients than venous PT. Otoscopic examination by a head and neck physician is essential to evaluate for possible ear pathologies such as middle ear fluid, cholesteatoma, or glomus tumor. In addition, fundoscopic examination to assess for optic disc edema could help to evaluate for idiopathic intracranial hypertension (IIH), a common cause of PT.

Imaging and Other Diagnostic Tests

For patients with isolated PT without other neurologic symptoms or with chronic symptoms, brain MRI with and without contrast in addition to magnetic resonance (MR) angiography and MR venography has a high sensitivity in identifying structural causes of PT.[6] For patients who present with PT in addition to severe headaches or acute visual changes or in the setting of trauma, a computed tomography (CT) of the head with CT angiography of the head and neck can serve as the initial imaging modality to evaluate for an acute process. If PT is persistent without an obvious etiology on CT, MRI should be considered next. Venous imaging with MR venography or CT venography allows for evaluation of asymmetry in the venous system, structural abnormalities, and patency of the vessels and should be obtained when evaluating for venous thrombosis or stenosis. In addition, high-resolution temporal bone CT imaging, which has a high sensitivity for identifying structural abnormalities that involve the auditory pathway, should be considered. Other neuroimaging modalities, such as high spatial resolution CT or dual-phase imaging, have been reported to be helpful in the workup of PT.[7]

Although noninvasive imaging has acceptable sensitivity for detecting structural and cerebrovascular causes of PT, it may miss more subtle findings. If clinical workup and imaging are suggestive of an underlying vascular cause, diagnostic cerebral angiography should be considered for further evaluation. Six-vessel diagnostic cerebral angiography should be the preferred method because arteriovenous pathologies often involve multiple vessels. Careful examination of the venous phase is essential. If the PT is suspected to be caused by venous sinus stenosis, cerebral venous manometry to measure venous sinus pressures and gradient may be needed to confirm the clinical suspicion and guide management. A gradient of greater than 8 mm Hg has been established as the threshold for endovascular intervention,[8] although this threshold has not been validated in prospective studies. Other studies have reported the use of a gradient of greater than 4 mm Hg as an indication for endovascular intervention when accompanied by symptoms.[9]

A balloon occlusion test can confirm a diagnosis of the cause of PT if an awake patient describes resolution of PT following balloon inflation across the lesion, and this confirmation can increase the likelihood of treatment success.[8]

When a patient's symptoms are suggestive of IIH, a lumbar puncture to test the cerebrospinal fluid (CSF) opening pressure is standard as part of the workup in addition to MRI.[10,11]

Notably, incidental findings on neuroimaging, especially of the venous system, are not uncommon. These incidental findings should only be further investigated with more advanced and invasive techniques if they are thought to be symptomatic or present a risk of hemorrhage to the patient.

Etiology of Pulsatile Tinnitus

Arterial causes of pulsatile tinnitus

PT can be caused by cervical carotid artery stenosis as a result of the turbulent flow across the carotid bifurcation due to plaque formation.[3] In these cases, carotid endarterectomy and carotid stenting have been described to improve PT[12]; however, the treatment of cervical carotid stenosis is typically reserved for symptomatic cases with high-grade stenosis (>70%). In patients with lower grade stenosis and with no history of transient ischemic attacks or stroke, medical optimization should be the first-line treatment.[13]

PT has also been linked to intracranial atherosclerotic disease, especially petrous carotid stenosis where the internal carotid artery courses within the temporal bone.[14] Medical management remains the primary treatment modality of intracranial atherosclerotic disease. In patients with high-grade stenosis and disabling PT, stenting has been reported to improve PT.[15] Likewise, petrous or cavernous carotid dissections with stenosis or pseudoaneurysm formation can result in PT.[16] If these injuries result in pseudoaneurysm formation, treatment may involve coiling, stent-assisted coiling, or flow diversion.[14]

PT may be caused by cervical carotid artery dissections in 5% to 15% of these patients,[17] and the

PT is often accompanied by other symptoms, including headache, neck pain, or neurologic deficits. These symptoms may occur spontaneously or after trauma. The usual first-line treatment involves antiplatelet or anticoagulation agents. Neither approach has been shown to have a higher efficacy than the other.[18] In the case of arterial dissection, PT tends to improve or resolve over the subsequent few months as the dissection heals. Medical treatment is often used for 3 to 6 months, and repeat CT angiography or MR angiography is obtained for follow-up. In patients who develop enlarging dissecting pseudoaneurysms, or high-grade stenosis and ischemic symptoms, stenting may be considered.[19]

Fibromuscular dysplasia with a "string-of-beads" appearance on imaging of the carotid arteries and steno-occlusive disease has been linked to PT, given the increased propensity with fibromuscular dysplasia for arterial stenosis, arterial dissections, and aneurysms.[20] Patients who have PT associated with fibromuscular dysplasia are treated with antiplatelet agents, and stenting is considered for cases with high-grade stenosis.[21] Intracranial aneurysms, although less common, have also been associated with PT given the focal region of turbulent flow.[22,23]

PT has also been linked to anatomic variants, including aberrant or ectopic internal carotid arteries,[24] carotid cochlear dehiscence,[25] an arterial vascular loop in the inner ear,[26] and a persistent stapedial artery.[27]

Venous causes of pulsatile tinnitus

Turbulent flow in the cerebral veins or venous sinuses can lead to PT.[9] Venous causes of PT tend to be more benign than arterial causes. Venous causes are typically related to sigmoid sinus diverticula, emissary vein anomalies (eg, a hypertrophied condylar vein), venous sinus stenosis or jugular vein anomalies (eg, a high-riding jugular bulb), or venous sinus thrombosis.[28] Patients with venous pathology may sometimes present with multiple anatomic abnormalities (eg, venous sinus stenosis and sigmoid wall malformations). Endovascular treatment of venous-related disorders has been performed with increased frequency.[28]

Venous sinus stenosis and idiopathic intracranial hypertension

Venous sinus stenosis is reported to cause PT by 1 of 2 mechanisms: increased velocity and turbulence of blood flow adjacent to the auditory pathway or through the effect of venous stenosis on CSF reabsorption.[9] The most common site of stenosis is at the junction of the transverse and sigmoid sinuses.[29] Transverse sinus stenosis can be related to a prominent arachnoid granulation that obstructs flow, septations, or thrombosis, or it can be the result of extrinsic compression (eg, high intracranial pressure, fracture, tumor).[30] The degree of stenosis can be highly variable and can range from mild asymmetry to near-complete occlusion.

IIH is associated with transverse/sigmoid sinus stenosis, but it is controversial whether the high CSF pressure collapses the sinus or, conversely, whether the venous outflow obstruction increases the CSF pressure.[9,31] IIH has an incidence of 20 per 100,000 in obese young females.[32] More than half of patients diagnosed with IIH report pulse-synchronous PT, and this may sometimes be the only symptom on presentation and may precede headaches and visual decline.[33] The modified Dandy diagnostic criteria for IIH include the presence of symptoms or signs of increased intracranial pressure, the absence of localizing examination findings, and the absence of intracranial lesions (except an empty sella sign).[10,11]

The first-line treatment for IIH typically includes weight loss and diet modification.[34] Acetazolamide, a carbonic anhydrase inhibitor that reduces the rate of CSF production, is often the first-line medication.[35] CSF shunting with a ventriculoperitoneal or a lumboperitoneal shunt, optic nerve sheath fenestration, and venous sinus stenting are considered for patients for whom medical treatment is unsuccessful, or in those who have adverse effects with acetazolamide or are who are noncompliant, and who have progressive headaches and impairment in visual acuity or constricted visual fields.[8,36,37] In patients with significant sinus stenosis, venous sinus stenting has been reported to have a high success rate for resolving PT (>90%) (**Fig. 1**).[38–40]

Venous sinus stenosis can be found without signs of increased intracranial pressure and can be an independent finding outside of the framework of IIH.[9] It most often occurs at the junction of the transverse and sigmoid sinuses, and it is typically unilateral. Stenosis of the sagittal sinus has also been described as a cause of PT, and it can occur spontaneously or associated with trauma or a fracture.[41] Venous sinus stenting has been used with high efficacy and low morbidity.[38–40] Recurrence of symptoms has been reported in 10% to 15% of cases and may be related to new stenosis adjacent to the stent or to in-stent stenosis.[8,42] Unlike arterial stents, the most common site of stenosis for stenting of the transverse/sigmoid sinus junction tends to be on the medial end of the transverse sinus.[43] Some interventionalists consider placing long stents or multiple stents to cross the medial end

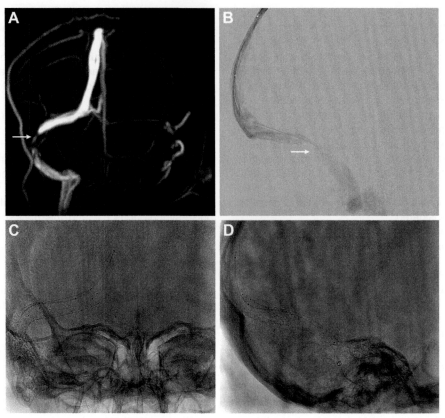

Fig. 1. A 26-year-old woman presented with headaches, pulsatile tinnitus, and worsening visual field deficits. Her examination was notable for papilledema. Findings from lumbar puncture were notable for elevated opening pressure. Her symptoms continued to worsen despite maximal medical management, including escalating doses of acetazolamide and attempted weight loss. (*A*) Magnetic resonance venography demonstrated a hypoplastic left transverse sinus and focal stenosis (*arrow*) of the lateral aspect of the right transverse sinus. (*B*) She underwent cerebral angiography and venography with venous sinus pressure measurement revealing a gradient of 20 mm Hg across the right transverse sinus stenosis (*arrow*). (*C* and *D*) After discussions of different treatment options, the patient underwent transverse sinus stenting. Procedure description: (*C*) Anteroposterior and (*D*) lateral views showing the right common femoral vein was accessed via the modified Seldinger technique under ultrasonographic visualization. A 7-F introducer sheath was then passed into the inferior vena cava. Next, a Benchmark BMX-81 guide catheter (Penumbra, Inc.) was advanced over a 5F Bernstein catheter and 0.038-inch diameter Glidewire and navigated into the right jugular bulb. The BMX catheter was eventually advanced into the sigmoid sinus. An Excelsior 1018 catheter (Stryker Neurovascular) was advanced over a 0.018-inch diameter Roadrunner exchange wire (Cook Medical) and these were navigated into the posterior third of the superior sagittal sinus. Then, a catheter exchange was performed, removing the Excelsior 1018 catheter and navigating an 8 × 40 mm Zilver biliary stent delivery device (Cook Medical) to the peritorcular region. The stent was then delivered, spanning the proximal right transverse sinus. Over the 0.018-inch diameter Roadrunner wire, a second 8 × 40 mm stent delivery device was then navigated in a telescoping fashion into the right transverse sinus stent, spanning the region of stenosis entirely. Used with permission from Barrow Neurological Institute, Phoenix, Arizona.

of the transverse sinus to prevent stent-adjacent-stenosis. Diagnostic cerebral angiography or CT venography should be obtained at 6 months for follow-up. If stenosis is accompanied by recurrence of the PT and is associated with a new venous gradient, placement of another stent may be considered. Patients are started on dual antiplatelet treatment typically for 3 to 6 months following stent placement and are subsequently maintained on aspirin. In patients who may not

be compliant, balloon angioplasty without stenting is a possible option but likely carries a higher rate of recurrence.[44]

Sigmoid sinus wall abnormalities
Sigmoid diverticula, sigmoid plate thinning, or dehiscence and sigmoid sinus ectasia are some of the most common causes of venous PT.[3,9,28] The right side, which is typically the dominant side, is more likely to be affected. In sigmoid sinus

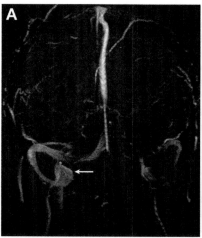 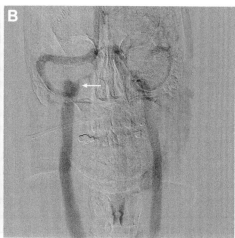

Fig. 2. A 73-year-old man presented for evaluation of persistent right-sided pulsatile tinnitus. (*A*) Magnetic resonance venography showed a high-riding right jugular bulb (*arrow*) and hypoplastic left transverse-sigmoid sinus. (*B*) Cerebral angiography also showed the high-riding jugular bulb (*arrow*) on the right. He was managed conservatively. Used with permission from Barrow Neurological Institute, Phoenix, Arizona.

diverticula, where an aneurysmal-like dilatation of the sigmoid sinus develops, coil embolization has been reported with a high success rate.[45,46] Like arterial aneurysms, the neck may be narrow or wide across the diverticulum. In diverticula with a wider neck, balloon-assisted or stent-assisted coiling techniques may be needed.[47]

In cases of sigmoid plate dehiscence where the overlying bone is absent or thinned, allowing for contact of the sigmoid sinus with the mastoid air cells, or sigmoid sinus ectasia where there is invasion into the mastoid air cells, surgical reconstruction of the sinus wall has been described using fat, muscle, or other agents.[48] However, these procedures may be associated with significant complications.[49] Stenting across the dehisced sinus could be another option.[9,48]

Transverse sinus stenosis is associated with a sigmoid sinus diverticulum and dehiscence, and some patients have both findings simultaneously; the turbulent flow across the stenosis is thought to promote poststenotic dilatation of the sigmoid sinus into a diverticular pouch.[50] In these cases, transverse sinus stenting or coiling of the sigmoid diverticulum has been used successfully.[9]

Jugular venous anomalies
A high-riding jugular bulb (**Fig. 2**), where the dome of the jugular bulb extends more superiorly into the petrous temporal bone than usual, has been implicated in PT, given the proximity to the cochlea.[51] On otoscopy, a hypotympanic blue lesion is noted.[28] The prevalence of a high-riding jugular bulb has been reported as between 6% and 34%.[52,53] A high-riding jugular bulb can also be associated with tympanic trauma or chronic ear

infections.[54] Endovascular options for an isolated, high-riding jugular bulb are limited, and surgical options have a high complication rate. Furthermore, stents placed across the jugular bulb may be associated with lower cranial nerve dysfunction, and stents in the jugular vein have a risk of migration.[53,55] A dehiscent high-riding jugular bulb can be associated with a diverticulum as well. Coil embolization of the diverticulum has been utilized in those cases.

Venous sinus thrombosis
Dural venous sinus thrombosis predominantly affects the sigmoid and transverse sinuses and can result in PT, which can be isolated or can be associated with headache, visual changes, or neurologic deficits.[56] It is encountered in patients with inherited or acquired coagulopathy, cancer, infection, or trauma. Severe cases of dural venous sinus thrombosis can result in intraparenchymal hemorrhage and increased intracranial pressure.[57] Anticoagulation is the treatment of choice for dural venous sinus thrombosis,[56] and it generally leads to resolution of PT over several months with recanalization of the sinus. Endovascular thrombectomy may be indicated in cases with progressive neurologic decline[58]; surgical decompression may be needed in cases of large or expanding intraparenchymal hemorrhage.[59] In patients with chronic residual sinus stenosis and disabling PT, stenting may be considered. Additionally, jugular venous thrombosis or stenosis can be implicated in PT.

Emissary vein abnormalities
Emissary veins are venous channels that connect the extracranial veins of the scalp to the intracranial

dural venous sinuses. Abnormalities of these channels can cause PT due to their proximity to the auditory pathways and most commonly involve the posterior condylar vein, the mastoid emissary vein, and the petrosquamosal vein.[3,9,28] The posterior condylar vein joins the jugular bulb with the deep cervical venous system. A dilated posterior condylar vein can be an isolated finding or can occur in the setting of internal jugular vein thrombosis or stenosis.[60] The mastoid emissary vein forms a transosseous connection between the sigmoid sinus and occipital veins that drain into the vertebral plexus. This emissary vein is present with high prevalence in the general population. In cases of stenosis of major outflow vessels, the mastoid vein can become dilated and can result in PT due to its course across the mastoid air cells (**Fig. 3**).[61,62] The petrosquamosal vein courses over the petrous bone and drains through several

pathways into the external jugular vein.[63] It usually disappears prenatally but may persist in some people.[64] When dilated, it can also result in PT. Coil embolization of these emissary veins has been reported; however, the venous anatomy must be carefully evaluated before embolization to avoid venous congestion and hemorrhage because these veins may sometimes serve as major outflow channels.[61,62,64]

Arteriovenous shunting

dAVFs occur most commonly at the transverse, sigmoid, or cavernous sinus (carotid-cavernous fistulas, **Fig. 4**) and can cause hemodynamic alterations resulting in PT.[65] The location of the fistulous connection, the presence of cortical venous drainage, and the direction of flow and presence of venous ectasia stratify the risk of dAVF and guide management.[66,67] If disabling

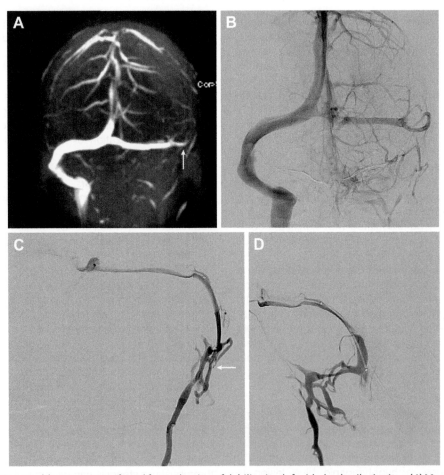

Fig. 3. A 59-year-old woman was referred for evaluation of debilitating left-sided pulsatile tinnitus. (*A*) Magnetic resonance angiography showed left sigmoid sinus occlusion (*arrow*). (*B*) Cerebral angiography was performed for further evaluation, again showing left sigmoid sinus occlusion. (*C*) Anteroposterior projection and (*D*) lateral projection views of selective microcatheterization of the left transverse sinus showed occlusion at the level of the left jugular bulb with a dilated mastoid vein (*arrow, C*). Used with permission from Barrow Neurological Institute, Phoenix, Arizona.

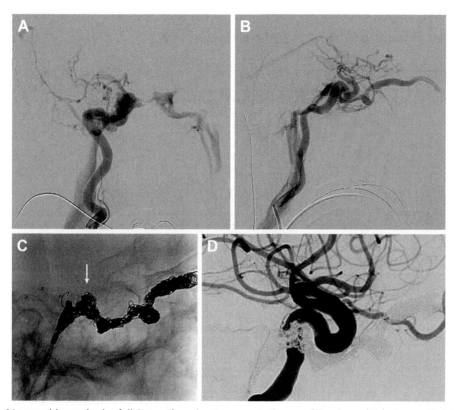

Fig. 4. A 64-year-old man had a fall 2 months prior to presentation resulting in multiple traumatic injuries. He later developed pulsatile tinnitus, followed by chemosis of his right eye, which prompted him to present for evaluation. (*A*) Anteroposterior and (*B*) lateral views of cerebral angiography showed a right-sided direct carotid cavernous fistula. The patient was treated endovascularly. Procedure description: Right radial arterial access and femoral venous access were obtained using the modified Seldinger technique under ultrasound guidance. A 7-F radial sheath and a 6-F femoral venous sheath were placed. A Benchmark BMX-81 guide catheter (Penumbra, Inc.) was navigated into the right internal carotid artery. An angled 6-French Envoy catheter was then navigated from the venous sheath into the right jugular bulb. An SL-10 microcatheter was then navigated into the posterior aspect of the superior ophthalmic vein, and coil embolization proceeded from anterior to posterior until the midsegment of the right cavernous sinus was reached. Next, through the BMX guide catheter in the right internal carotid artery, a CAT 5 catheter (Stryker), Phenom 27 microcatheter (Medtronic), and Synchro 0.014-inch diameter guidewire (Stryker) were advanced into the right supraclinoid internal carotid artery, and (*C*) a Pipeline embolization device (Medtronic) (*arrow*) was deployed, covering the fistulous connection. Following that, additional transvenous embolization was performed from the midsegment of the cavernous sinus into the posterior aspect with coils and Onyx-18 (Medtronic) occluding the posterior aspect of the right cavernous sinus and the inferior petrosal sinus. (*D*) This procedure resulted in complete obliteration of the carotid cavernous fistula with no additional shunting. Used with permission from Barrow Neurological Institute, Phoenix, Arizona.

PT is present in a lesion with high-risk features, treatment is recommended. In benign lesions, where the risk of hemorrhage is low, conservative management should be the strategy of choice.[66,67] However, if PT is severe and affects the activities of daily living in these patients, endovascular intervention can be considered. The usual management of dAVFs involves cerebral angiography and endovascular embolization with liquid embolic agents (Onyx or nBCA) or coiling through transarterial or transvernous approaches.[68] There is a high rate of PT resolution with occlusion of the fistula.[69]

Other causes of pulsatile tinnitus

Tumors, most commonly vestibular schwannomas and paragangliomas, and temporal bone pathologies result in alterations in the inner ear with increased bone conduction causing the normal flow sounds in the body to be perceived more intensely.[2] Combined neurosurgical and otolaryngologic approaches have high safety and efficacy for these pathologies (**Table 1**).

Nonoperative Management

Notably, nonoperative interventions focused on behavioral changes and coping skills have also

Table 1
Etiology and associated treatment options for pulsatile tinnitus

Pathology	Treatment Options
Arterial	
Cerebral aneurysms	Radiographic surveillance, endovascular treatment, or microsurgical clipping depending on patient and aneurysm factors
Arterial dissection (cervical or petrous/cavernous) with or without pseudoaneurysm	Medical management with antiplatelet or anticoagulation agents. Coiling, stenting, stent-assisted coiling, or flow diversion for enlarging, symptomatic pseudoaneurysms
Cervical atherosclerotic disease with associated stenosis	Medical management with antiplatelet agents, statins, blood pressure control or intervention (carotid artery stenting or carotid endarterectomy), depending on symptomatology and degree of stenosis
Intracranial atherosclerotic disease (most commonly petrous)	Medical management primarily; stenting may be indicated if severe or recurrent symptoms are present
Fibromuscular dysplasia	Medical management with antiplatelet agents; stenting in cases of severe, symptomatic stenosis

Anatomic variants
  Aberrant internal carotid artery
  Carotid cochlear dehiscence
  Arterial vascular loop in the inner ear
  Persistent stapedial artery
	Observation and medical management. Endovascular treatment for vessel occlusion is rarely indicated. Endoscopic ear surgery and microvascular decompression techniques have been described in cases with debilitating PT

Venous	
Idiopathic intracranial hypertension	Medical management with weight loss and acetazolamide. CSF shunting, venous sinus stenting, or optic nerve sheath fenestration in cases refractory to medical management
Venous sinus stenosis unrelated to idiopathic intracranial hypertension	Venous sinus stenting in symptomatic cases with a high pressure gradient across the stenosis.
Sigmoid sinus diverticulum	Coiling, balloon-assisted coiling, or stent-assisted coiling
Sigmoid plate thinning/dehiscence and sigmoid sinus ectasia	Medical management. Surgical reconstruction of the sinus wall or endovascular stenting, rarely
High-riding jugular bulb	Often treated conservatively. Surgical reconstructive options and endovascular stenting, rarely
Venous sinus thrombosis	Anticoagulation in the acute setting. Endovascular thrombectomy in severe or refractory cases. Stenting in cases with residual stenosis

Emissary vein abnormalities
  Posterior condylar vein
  Mastoid emissary vein
  Petrosquamosal vein
	Coil embolization of the emissary vein

Arterio-venous shunting	
Transverse-sigmoid sinus dural arteriovenous fistula (dAVF) Carotid-cavernous sinus dAVF Super sagittal sinus dAVF	Endovascular embolization with liquid embolic agents (Onyx or nBCA) or coiling through transarterial or transvernous approaches. Observation for low-grade lesions without cortical venous drainage

Tumor/otologic
  Vestibular schwannomas
  Paragangliomas
  Temporal bone pathologies
	Microsurgical resection or repair through combined neurosurgical and otolaryngologic approaches

been used for PT and may be an option for patients who do not have abnormal structural findings on workup, patients with benign pathologies, and patients who do not want to undergo an endovascular or surgical intervention.[70] Tinnitus retraining therapy and cognitive behavioral therapy to provide coping skills have been described.[2,71]

SUMMARY

PT requires detailed workup. Venous causes of PT are among the most common structural pathologies causing this symptom and may warrant intervention. Careful evaluation of the venous sinuses, jugular bulb, and emissary veins on noninvasive vascular imaging and cerebral angiography can lead to identification of the underlying cause and guide treatment. Endovascular tools have proven safety and efficacy in the management of venous causes of PT, but these results have primarily derived from institutional case reports and case series. As our understanding of these venous anomalies grows, more standardized protocols and future trials are needed to guide contemporary practice.

CLINICS CARE POINTS

- Pulsatile tinnitus can be associated with cerebrovascular arterial or venous pathologies and requires clinical evaluation.
- Venous causes of pulsatile tinnitus are becoming increasingly recognized, and endovascular treatment options have demonstrated high safety and efficacy in addressing these lesions.
- Careful evaluation of the venous sinuses, jugular bulb, and emissary veins on noninvasive vascular imaging and cerebral angiography can lead to identification of the underlying cause and guide treatment.

FINANCIAL SUPPORT

None.

ACKNOWLEDGMENTS

The authors thank the staff of Neuroscience Publications at Barrow Neurological Institute for assistance with manuscript preparation.

DISCLOSURE

Dr A.F. Ducruet is a consultant for Stryker, Medtronic, Cerenovus, Koswire, Penumbra, Inc., Balt, and Phenox and has ownership interest in Aneuvas Technologies, Inc. Dr B.J. Daou has no personal, financial, or institutional interest in any of the drugs, materials, or devices described in this article.

REFERENCES

1. Jarach CM, Lugo A, Scala M, et al. Global prevalence and incidence of tinnitus: a systematic review and meta-analysis. JAMA Neurol 2022;79(9):888–900.
2. Narsinh KH, Hui F, Saloner D, et al. Diagnostic approach to pulsatile tinnitus: a narrative review. JAMA Otolaryngol Head Neck Surg 2022;148(5):476–83.
3. Narsinh KH, Hui F, Duvvuri M, et al. Management of vascular causes of pulsatile tinnitus. J Neurointerventional Surg 2022;14(11):1151–7.
4. Cummins DD, Caton MT, Hemphill K, et al. Clinical evaluation of pulsatile tinnitus: history and physical examination techniques to predict vascular etiology. J Neurointerventional Surg 2023. https://doi.org/10.1136/jnis-2023-020440.
5. Hofmann E, Behr R, Neumann-Haefelin T, et al. Pulsatile tinnitus: imaging and differential diagnosis. Dtsch Arztebl Int 2013;110(26):451–8.
6. Pegge SAH, Steens SCA, Kunst HPM, et al. Pulsatile tinnitus: differential diagnosis and radiological workup. Curr Radiol Rep 2017;5(1):5.
7. Krishnan A, Mattox DE, Fountain AJ, et al. CT arteriography and venography in pulsatile tinnitus: preliminary results. AJNR Am J Neuroradiol 2006;27(8):1635–8.
8. Ahmed RM, Wilkinson M, Parker GD, et al. Transverse sinus stenting for idiopathic intracranial hypertension: a review of 52 patients and of model predictions. AJNR Am J Neuroradiol 2011;32(8):1408–14.
9. Abdalkader M, Nguyen TN, Norbash AM, et al. State of the art: Venous causes of pulsatile tinnitus and diagnostic considerations guiding endovascular therapy. Radiology 2021;300(1):2–16.
10. Dandy WE. Intracranial pressure without brain tumor: diagnosis and treatment. Ann Surg 1937;106(4):492–513.
11. Smith JL. Whence pseudotumor cerebri? J Clin Neuro Ophthalmol 1985;5(1):55–6.
12. Kirkby-Bott J, Gibbs HH. Carotid endarterectomy relieves pulsatile tinnitus associated with severe ipsilateral carotid stenosis. Eur J Vasc Endovasc Surg 2004;27(6):651–3.
13. Ferguson GG, Eliasziw M, Barr HW, et al. The North American Symptomatic Carotid Endarterectomy Trial: surgical results in 1415 patients. Stroke 1999;30(9):1751–8.
14. Pingree GM, Fleming C, Reavey-Cantwell J, et al. Neurosurgical causes of pulsatile tinnitus: contemporary update. Neurosurgery 2022;90(2):161–9.

15. Ihn YK, Jung WS, Kim BS. Disappeared pulsatile tinnitus related to petrous segment stenosis of the ICA after relief of the stenosis by stenting. Intervent Neuroradiol 2013;19(1):97–101.

16. Pelkonen O, Tikkakoski T, Luotonen J, et al. Pulsatile tinnitus as a symptom of cervicocephalic arterial dissection. J Laryngol Otol 2004;118(3):193–8.

17. Chen SY, Zipfel GJ, Wick CC. Internal carotid artery dissection causing pulsatile tinnitus. Am J Otolaryngol 2019;40(1):121–3.

18. Daou B, Hammer C, Mouchtouris N, et al. Anticoagulation vs antiplatelet treatment in patients with carotid and vertebral artery dissection: a study of 370 patients and literature review. Neurosurgery 2017; 80(3):368–79.

19. Daou B, Hammer C, Chalouhi N, et al. Dissecting pseudoaneurysms: predictors of symptom occurrence, enlargement, clinical outcome, and treatment. J Neurosurg 2016;125(4):936–42.

20. Dicks AB, Gornik HL, Gu X, et al. Association of fibromuscular dysplasia and pulsatile tinnitus: a report of the US Registry for Fibromuscular Dysplasia. J Am Heart Assoc 2021;10(17):e021962.

21. Wells RP, Smith RR. Fibromuscular dysplasia of the internal carotid artery: a long term follow-up. Neurosurgery 1982;10(1):39–43.

22. Kim DK, Shin YS, Lee JH, et al. Pulsatile tinnitus as the sole manifestation of an internal carotid artery aneurysm successfully treated by coil embolization. Clin Exp Otorhinolaryngol 2012;5(3):170–2.

23. Kim SM, Kim CH, Lee CY. Petrous carotid aneurysm causing pulsatile tinnitus: case report and review of the literature. J Cerebrovasc Endovasc Neurosurg 2018;20(1):35–9.

24. Song YS, Yuan YY, Wang GJ, et al. Aberrant internal carotid artery causing objective pulsatile tinnitus and conductive hearing loss. Acta Otolaryngol 2012;132(10):1126–30.

25. Lund AD, Palacios SD. Carotid artery-cochlear dehiscence: a review. Laryngoscope 2011;121(12): 2658–60.

26. De Ridder D, De Ridder L, Nowe V, et al. Pulsatile tinnitus and the intrameatal vascular loop: why do we not hear our carotids? Neurosurgery 2005; 57(6):1213–7 [discussion: 1213-7].

27. Goderie TPM, Alkhateeb WHF, Smit CF, et al. Surgical management of a persistent stapedial artery: a review. Otol Neurotol 2017;38(6):788–91.

28. Essibayi MA, Oushy SH, Lanzino G, et al. Venous causes of pulsatile tinnitus: clinical presentation, clinical and radiographic evaluation, pathogenesis, and endovascular treatments: a literature review. Neurosurgery 2021;89(5):760–8.

29. Raz E, Nossek E, Jethanamest D, et al. Emergence of venous stenosis as the dominant cause of pulsatile tinnitus. Stroke Vasc Interv Neurol 2022;2(4): e000154.

30. Strydom MA, Briers N, Bosman MC, et al. The anatomical basis of venographic filling defects of the transverse sinus. Clin Anat 2010;23(2):153–9.

31. Farb RI, Vanek I, Scott JN, et al. Idiopathic intracranial hypertension: the prevalence and morphology of sinovenous stenosis. Neurology 2003;60(9): 1418–24.

32. Radhakrishnan K, Thacker AK, Bohlaga NH, et al. Epidemiology of idiopathic intracranial hypertension: a prospective and case-control study. J Neurol Sci 1993;116(1):18–28.

33. Giuseffi V, Wall M, Siegel PZ, et al. Symptoms and disease associations in idiopathic intracranial hypertension (pseudotumor cerebri): a case-control study. Neurology 1991;41(2):239–44. Pt 1.

34. Johnson LN, Krohel GB, Madsen RW, et al. The role of weight loss and acetazolamide in the treatment of idiopathic intracranial hypertension (pseudotumor cerebri). Ophthalmology 1998;105(12):2313–7.

35. Committee NIIHSGW, Wall M, McDermott MP, et al. Effect of acetazolamide on visual function in patients with idiopathic intracranial hypertension and mild visual loss: the idiopathic intracranial hypertension treatment trial. JAMA 2014;311(16):1641–51.

36. Banta JT, Farris BK. Pseudotumor cerebri and optic nerve sheath decompression. Ophthalmology 2000; 107(10):1907–12.

37. Sweid A, Daou BJ, Weinberg JH, et al. Experience with ventriculoperitoneal and lumboperitoneal shunting for the treatment of idiopathic intracranial hypertension: a single institution series. Oper Neurosurg (Hagerstown) 2021;21(2):57–62.

38. Boddu S, Dinkin M, Suurna M, et al. Resolution of pulsatile tinnitus after venous sinus stenting in patients with idiopathic intracranial hypertension. PLoS One 2016;11(10):e0164466.

39. Nicholson P, Brinjikji W, Radovanovic I, et al. Venous sinus stenting for idiopathic intracranial hypertension: a systematic review and meta-analysis. J Neurointerventional Surg 2019;11(4):380–5.

40. Lim J, Monteiro A, Kuo CC, et al. Stenting for venous sinus stenosis in patients with idiopathic intracranial hypertension: an updated systematic review and meta-analysis of the literature. Neurosurgery 2023.

41. Zabalo San Juan G, Vazquez Miguez A, Zazpe Cenoz I, et al. Intracranial hypertension caused by superior sagittal sinus stenosis secondary to a depressed skull fracture: case report and review of the literature. Neurocirugia (Astur: Engl Ed). Sep-Oct 2019;30(5):243–9.

42. Garner RM, Aldridge JB, Wolfe SQ, et al. Quality of life, need for retreatment, and the re-equilibration phenomenon after venous sinus stenting for idiopathic intracranial hypertension. J Neurointerventional Surg 2021; 13(1):79–85.

43. Fargen KM. A unifying theory explaining venous sinus stenosis and recurrent stenosis following

venous sinus stenting in patients with idiopathic intracranial hypertension. J Neurointerventional Surg 2021;13(7):587–92.

44. Carlos Martinez-Gutierrez J, Kole MJ, Lopez-Rivera V, et al. Primary balloon angioplasty of venous sinus stenosis in idiopathic intracranial hypertension. Intervent Neuroradiol 2023;29(4): 358–62.

45. Mehanna R, Shaltoni H, Morsi H, et al. Endovascular treatment of sigmoid sinus aneurysm presenting as devastating pulsatile tinnitus. A case report and review of literature. Intervent Neuroradiol 2010;16(4): 451–4.

46. Park YH, Kwon HJ. Awake embolization of sigmoid sinus diverticulum causing pulsatile tinnitus: simultaneous confirmative diagnosis and treatment. Intervent Neuroradiol 2011;17(3):376–9.

47. Paramasivam S, Furtado S, Shigamatsu T, et al. Endovascular management of sigmoid sinus diverticulum. Interv Neurol 2016;5(1–2):76–80.

48. Eisenman DJ. Sinus wall reconstruction for sigmoid sinus diverticulum and dehiscence: a standardized surgical procedure for a range of radiographic findings. Otol Neurotol 2011;32(7):1116–9.

49. Eisenman DJ, Raghavan P, Hertzano R, et al. Evaluation and treatment of pulsatile tinnitus associated with sigmoid sinus wall anomalies. Laryngoscope 2018;128(Suppl 2):S1–13.

50. Han Y, Yang Q, Yang Z, et al. Computational fluid dynamics simulation of hemodynamic alterations in sigmoid sinus diverticulum and ipsilateral upstream sinus stenosis after stent implantation in patients with pulsatile tinnitus. World Neurosurg 2017;106: 308–14.

51. Kao E, Kefayati S, Amans MR, et al. Flow patterns in the jugular veins of pulsatile tinnitus patients. J Biomech 2017;52:61–7.

52. Aksoy SH, Yurdaisik I. High riding jugular bulb: prevalence and significance in asymptomatic children. Acta Radiol 2023;64(2):792–7.

53. Manjila S, Bazil T, Kay M, et al. Jugular bulb and skull base pathologies: proposal for a novel classification system for jugular bulb positions and microsurgical implications. Neurosurg Focus 2018;45(1): E5.

54. Kondoh K, Kitahara T, Mishiro Y, et al. Management of hemorrhagic high jugular bulb with adhesive otitis media in an only hearing ear: transcatheter endovascular embolization using detachable coils. Ann Otol Rhinol Laryngol 2004;113(12):975–9.

55. Couloigner V, Grayeli AB, Bouccara D, et al. Surgical treatment of the high jugular bulb in patients with Meniere's disease and pulsatile tinnitus. Eur Arch Oto-Rhino-Laryngol 1999;256(5):224–9.

56. Saposnik G, Barinagarrementeria F, Brown RD, et al. Diagnosis and management of cerebral venous thrombosis. Stroke 2011;42(4):1158–92.

57. Wasay M, Bakshi R, Bobustuc G, et al. Cerebral venous thrombosis: analysis of a multicenter cohort from the United States. J Stroke Cerebrovasc Dis 2008;17(2):49–54.

58. Stam J, Majoie CB, van Delden OM, et al. Endovascular thrombectomy and thrombolysis for severe cerebral sinus thrombosis: a prospective study. Stroke 2008;39(5):1487–90.

59. Coutinho JM, Majoie CB, Coert BA, et al. Decompressive hemicraniectomy in cerebral sinus thrombosis: consecutive case series and review of the literature. Stroke 2009;40(6):2233–5.

60. Lambert PR, Cantrell RW. Objective tinnitus in association with an abnormal posterior condylar emissary vein. Am J Otol 1986;7(3):204–7.

61. Abdalkader M, Ma A, Cohen M, et al. Endovascular coiling of large mastoid emissary vein causing pulsatile tinnitus. Intervent Neuroradiol 2020;26(6): 821–5.

62. Eliezer M, Freitas RK, Fantoni M, et al. Selective embolization of the mastoid emissary vein for pulsatile tinnitus treatment: when is it indicated? J Neurointerventional Surg 2020;12(10):999–1001.

63. Marsot-Dupuch K, Gayet-Delacroix M, Elmaleh-Berges M, et al. The petrosquamosal sinus: CT and MR findings of a rare emissary vein. AJNR Am J Neuroradiol 2001;22(6):1186–93.

64. Mortazavi MM, Tubbs RS, Riech S, et al. Anatomy and pathology of the cranial emissary veins: a review with surgical implications. Neurosurgery 2012; 70(5):1312–8 [discussion 1318-9].

65. An YH, Han S, Lee M, et al. Dural arteriovenous fistula masquerading as pulsatile tinnitus: radiologic assessment and clinical implications. Sci Rep 2016;6:36601.

66. Borden JA, Wu JK, Shucart WA. A proposed classification for spinal and cranial dural arteriovenous fistulous malformations and implications for treatment. J Neurosurg 1995;82(2):166–79.

67. Cognard C, Gobin YP, Pierot L, et al. Cerebral dural arteriovenous fistulas: clinical and angiographic correlation with a revised classification of venous drainage. Radiology 1995;194(3):671–80.

68. Baharvahdat H, Ooi YC, Kim WJ, et al. Updates in the management of cranial dural arteriovenous fistula. Stroke Vasc Neurol 2020;5(1):50–8.

69. Delgado F, Munoz F, Bravo-Rodriguez F, et al. Treatment of dural arteriovenous fistulas presenting as pulsatile tinnitus. Otol Neurotol 2009;30(7):897–902.

70. Cima RF, Maes IH, Joore MA, et al. Specialised treatment based on cognitive behaviour therapy versus usual care for tinnitus: a randomised controlled trial. Lancet 2012;379(9830):1951–9.

71. Hesser H, Weise C, Westin VZ, et al. A systematic review and meta-analysis of randomized controlled trials of cognitive-behavioral therapy for tinnitus distress. Clin Psychol Rev 2011;31(4):545–53.

Cavernous Sinus Thrombosis

Steven B. Housley, MD, MS[a,b], Matthew J. McPheeters, MD, MBA[a,b], Kunal P. Raygor, MD[a,b], Mehdi Bouslama, MD, MSc[a,b], Tyler Scullen, MD[a,b], Jason M. Davies, MD, PhD[a,b,c,d,e,*]

KEYWORDS

- Cavernous sinus • Thrombosis • Venous sinus thrombosis • Cavernous sinus syndrome
- Danger triangle

KEY POINTS

- Cavernous sinus thrombosis is a rare but potentially lethal disease.
- Patients with this disease can present with meningitic symptoms, proptosis, chemosis, pyrexia, cranial nerve deficits, papilledema, vision loss, severe lethargy, and/or coma.
- Cavernous sinus thrombosis may occur secondary to septic and aseptic etiologies.
- Risk factors include infection of the "danger triangle," neoplasia, hormone-replacement therapy, pregnancy, thrombophilic disorders, and trauma.
- Treatment depends on the etiology and symptomatology and may involve antibiotics, anticoagulation, corticosteroids, and surgery.

INTRODUCTION

Cavernous sinus thrombosis (CST), a subset of cerebral sinus thrombosis, is a rare, but potentially life-threatening, condition that involves the formation of a thrombus within the cavernous sinus (CS). The annual incidence of CST is estimated to be 0.2 to 1.6 per 100,000 persons.[1] Although cerebral sinus thrombosis generally exhibits a female predominance, with up to 75% of those affected being women in the adult population and a near-equal gender distribution in pediatric and geriatric populations, CST appears to have an overall slight male predominance.[2,3] Because of its infrequent presentation, prognostication can be difficult; however, mortality rates have steadily declined with time. Recent estimates of morbidity and mortality are approximately 15% and 11%, respectively.[3]

The clinical features of CST are related to the unique anatomy and physiology of the CS, which contains portions of the internal carotid artery, oculomotor nerve (cranial nerve [CN] III), trochlear nerve (CN IV), trigeminal nerve (CN V1 and V2), and the abducens nerve (CN VI).[4,5] Additionally, the CS collects venous blood from the superior and inferior ophthalmic veins, sphenoid sinus, and the superficial cortical vein before draining via the superior and inferior petrosal sinuses and the pterygoid venous plexus (**Fig. 1**).[4] Communication between the bilateral CSs occurs between the anterior, inferior, and posterior interCSs and the basilar sinus.[5] Because of these extensive interconnections, symptoms associated with CST vary and include headache, pyrexia, ocular pain, proptosis, chemosis, periorbital edema, and CN palsies secondary to direct compression or irritation within the CS.[6] Clinicians must remain vigilant in diagnosing CST because it has the potential to rapidly become lethal.

[a] Department of Neurosurgery, Jacobs School of Medicine and Biomedical Sciences, University at Buffalo, 100 High Street, Suite B4, Buffalo, NY 14203, USA; [b] Department of Neurosurgery, Jacobs School of Medicine and Biomedical Sciences, University at Buffalo, Buffalo, NY 14201, USA; [c] Department of Bioinformatics, Jacobs School of Medicine and Biomedical Sciences, University at Buffalo, Buffalo, NY, USA; [d] Canon Stroke and Vascular Research Center, University at Buffalo, Buffalo, NY, USA; [e] Jacobs Institute, Buffalo, NY, USA
* Corresponding author. University at Buffalo Neurosurgery, 100 High Street, Suite B4, Buffalo, NY 14203.
E-mail address: jdavies@ubns.com

Neurosurg Clin N Am 35 (2024) 305–310
https://doi.org/10.1016/j.nec.2024.02.002
1042-3680/24/© 2024 Elsevier Inc. All rights reserved.

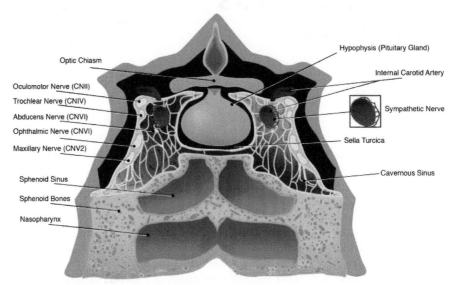

Fig. 1. Anatomy of the cavernous sinus. CN, cranial nerve. ("File:Anatomy of the cavernous sinus.jpg" by Okkes Kuybu, MD and Diana is licensed under CC BY 4.0. To view a copy of this license, visit https://creativecommons.org/licenses/by/4.0/?ref=openverse.)

DISCUSSION
Etiology

CST most commonly results from septic etiologies. These include sinusitis, otitis, erysipelas, mastoiditis, and odontogenic and facial infections.[7] In fact, most cases (60%–80%) arise from infection of the middle third of the face in what is known as the "danger triangle"[5,8] (**Fig. 2**). Ethmoid and sphenoid sinusitis represent more than 50% of the sources, middle ear infections are estimated to cause 10%, and both oral and dental infections have been estimated to represent less than 10% of cases.[5] *Staphylococcus aureus* is the most common microorganism, accounting for approximately 66% to 70% of cases.[5,7] *Streptococcus* species (20%), oral anaerobic flora (10%), and gram-negative bacteria (5%) may also be involved.[5] Less commonly, fungal etiologies, such as aspergillosis, mucormycosis, and actinomycosis, and/or viral etiologies have been reported.[5,9]

Despite the preponderance of septic causes, aseptic cases do occur. For instance, trauma and surgery to the head and neck region may lead to CST. Thrombophilic disorders, such as factor V Leiden mutation, myeloproliferative disorders, antiphospholipid syndrome, prothrombin G20210 A mutation, hyperhomocysteinemia, protein C and/or S resistance or deficiencies, and antithrombin deficiencies, have also been associated with CST.[2] Neoplasia, both local and metastatic, has been reported. Tumors in the CS region are most commonly cancers of the head and neck as well as pituitary adenomas, cavernous meningiomas, cavernous hemangiomas, and neurogenic tumors of the cranial CNs within the CS. More uncommonly, metastases from the breast and lung and prostate cancer have been reported.[9,10] Lymphomas have also

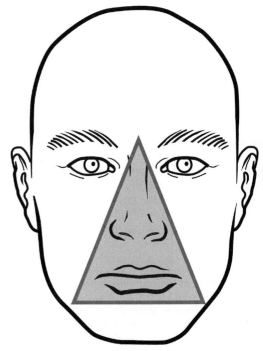

Fig. 2. Diagram illustrating the "danger triangle" of the face. (*Courtesy* of Paul H. Dressel BFA) (no permission required)

been reported to be involved.[11–14] Finally, hormone-based oral contraceptives, hormone-replacement therapies, and pregnancy have also been associated with CST.[2,5,7,15,16]

Differential Diagnosis

Early in the course of CST, nonspecific symptoms, such as pyrexia, headache, emesis, and signs of meningeal irritation, may lead to a mistaken diagnosis of meningitis. Because CST and meningitis often coexist, appropriate evaluation and potential treatment of meningitis should be performed.[5,17] In septic CST, lumbar puncture will often demonstrate an inflammatory profile, yet cerebrospinal fluid cultures are negative approximately 20% of the time.[5]

Orbital cellulitis and superior orbital fissure syndrome may both present in a very similar manner to CST. Patients who have orbital cellulitis may experience periorbital swelling, chemosis, proptosis, diplopia, and reduced visual acuity. This infection is often unilateral and not associated with papilledema, pupillary changes, or systemic toxic symptoms.[5] Superior orbital fissure syndrome is characterized by external ophthalmoplegia, exophthalmos, and Horner's syndrome or orbital apex syndrome (when visual impairment is present).[5] Patients with orbital apex syndrome classically present with visual loss and ophthalmoplegia that are out of proportion to and/or precede signs of orbital inflammation, such as periorbital edema, proptosis, and chemosis.[18]

CS syndrome may also be mistaken for CST because it is characterized by multiple cranial neuropathies, Horner's syndrome, and either hyperesthesia or hypoesthesia of the trigeminal nerve.[9,10] Oculosympathetic and oculoparasympathetic effects to the pupil may or may not be present in CS syndrome.[10] Specific CNs involved include the oculomotor nerve, trochlear nerve, the ophthalmic and maxillary divisions of the trigeminal nerve, and the abducens nerve. Multiple etiologies of CS syndrome exist, such as primary or metastatic neoplasia, granulomatous inflammation (ie, Tolosa-Hunt syndrome), cavernous carotid fistula, and cavernous carotid aneurysm, all of which lead to local compression of CS contents.[5,10] Multiple etiologies listed earlier may also contribute to CS syndrome and are not exclusive to CST.

Evaluation

Patients with CST may present with a multitude of symptoms, including headache (52%–90% of cases), pyrexia (90% of cases), nuchal rigidity (40% of cases), periorbital and facial hyperesthesia or hypoesthesia and swelling, chemosis, proptosis, photophobia, diplopia, painful extraocular movement, ophthalmoplegia (50%–80% of cases), papilledema, loss of corneal reflex, retinal venous distention, and vision loss (8%–15% of cases).[5,16,19] Severe cases often present with prominent symptoms of sepsis including tachycardia, emesis, hypotension, confusion, rigors, and even coma.[5] Pyrexia associated with CST is characterized by a "picket fence" pattern with high spikes followed by normothermia, suggestive of thrombophlebitis.[17] Symptoms are often initially present unilaterally; however, they may progress bilaterally without appropriate treatment as the infection and thrombosis spread through the interCSs. Special consideration is warranted in patients with the aforementioned etiologies and those who are immunocompromised secondary to conditions such as diabetes, long-term corticosteroid use, chronic alcohol or drug abuse, human immunodeficiency virus or acquired immunodeficiency syndrome, or bone marrow transplantation.[4]

There are no specific laboratory diagnostic tests for CST, but the test results may help establish the etiology, causative microorganism, or both. Patients are often found to have marked elevations in polymorphonuclear leukocytes, erythrocyte sedimentation rate, C-reactive protein, and D-dimer.[20–22] In cases of septic CST, identification of the causative microorganism can help guide and focus treatment. In most cases, cultures of the primary infective source, blood, and concurrent suppurations yield positive results.[5] A lumbar puncture may be an appropriate diagnostic test when concurrent signs of meningoencephalitis are present. When performed, 82% to 100% of patients will demonstrate an inflammatory profile indicative of bacterial infection; however, cultures are only positive in approximately 20% of cases.[5]

Imaging

Although a diagnosis of CST is often possible from clinical symptoms alone, improvements in imaging modalities have enabled early diagnosis and improved surveillance. Various venographic techniques of magnetic resonance (MR) and computed tomography (CT) imaging are used to evaluate for venous thrombi.[23] Two-dimensional, unenhanced time-of-flight MR venography is often employed; this technique exhibits excellent sensitivity to slow flow and diminished sensitivity to signal loss from saturation effects as compared to 3-dimensional counterparts.[23] Additionally, contrast-enhanced MR venography with elliptical centric view-ordering has been applied to improve visual resolution of small vessels and venous sinuses.[23,24] CT venography is often used due to being more readily available and the speed at which imaging can be completed. It is approximately 95% sensitive for detecting venous sinus thrombosis when multiplanar reformatted images are employed.[25] In fact, the detail of most CT venography images is superior to that of MR venography, albeit with some technical difficulties relating to reduction of bony artifact without losing contrast signal within the adjacent sinus.[23,25] This bony artifact is especially prominent in CST because the CS lies along the skull base. Additional imaging modalities, including nonenhanced T2 MR sequences where anomalies may be present within the venous flow voids and nonenhanced CT imaging where hyperdensities may be seen along the course of the sinuses, may be utilized in the absence of the more optimal imaging mentioned earlier.

Regardless of the imaging modality performed, both direct and indirect radiographic signs should be used to confirm the diagnosis.[5] Direct signs include expansion or filling defects within the CS. In several studies, bulging of the lateral wall was found to be the most frequent and sensitive sign associated with CST.[26,27] Asymmetric filling between the paired CSs confirmed the diagnosis.[28] Indirect signs of CST include narrowing or occlusion of the intracavernous portion of the internal carotid artery, reversal of normal venous flow at the skull base, increased dural enhancement at the CS border, exophthalmos, fat pad edema, or secondary thrombosis of the superior ophthalmic vein, or petrosal, sphenoparietal, or sigmoid sinus.[5,26,27] Additional indirect signs include venous dilation, restricted diffusion, or thickening of the superior ophthalmic veins.[5] Despite the signs listed earlier, the imaging findings may be normal early in the disease; therefore, empiric treatment is warranted when a high index of clinical suspicion exists.

Therapeutic Options

Although no randomized trial results exist to guide treatments for CST, likely due to the sparsity of the disease, many investigators have reported on their experience and expert opinions on optimal treatment algorithms. At present, patient stabilization, resuscitation, and management of the underlying etiology are paramount.[17] Management of the primary etiology may include appropriate antibiotics, anticoagulation, corticosteroids, and surgery.

Certainly, antibiotics have had the greatest impact on the prognosis of CST, especially because most cases are septic in nature and the associated mortality has been reduced in the antibiotic era.[3,17] Empiric antibiotic regimens should be initiated as soon as possible based on the most likely pathogens involved, which depends on the suspected infectious origin.[7] Appropriate empiric regimens include a third-generation cephalosporin (ie, ceftriaxone, cefotaxime, ceftazidime), metronidazole, and nafcillin or vancomycin.[5,7,29] Antibiotic therapy may be guided once culture and sensitivity testing results are available. Antifungals are rarely necessary unless the patient is immunocompromised or has a history of poorly controlled diabetes.[5] Antibiotics should be administered for a minimum duration of 3 to 4 weeks, consistent with the management of other intravascular infections, such as endotheliitis and suppurative phlebitis.[29]

Corticosteroids have been investigated for the treatment of CST; however, no consensus has been established. Proposed benefits include decreased orbital and CN inflammation as well as decreased vasogenic edema.[5] Weerasinghe and Lueck[3] performed a literature review in 2016 in 88 patients with CST and found no significant improvements associated with corticosteroid therapy among patients who achieved full recovery, survived with disability, or died. Additionally, Canhao and colleagues[30] reported on the use of corticosteroids in dural venous thrombosis and demonstrated no evidence of improvement to support steroid use. Nonetheless, steroids may prove useful in patients who have adrenal insufficiency or pituitary dysfunction secondary to the disease.[7] Ultimately, the potential benefits of corticosteroids must be weighed against their potential immunosuppressive effects and prothrombotic properties.[31]

Anticoagulation, a mainstay of dural venous sinus thrombosis, remains controversial in the treatment of CST; however, in their literature review of CST patients, Weerasinghe and Lueck[3] found that anticoagulated patients had a considerably greater rate of full recovery (53.6% vs 32%) and fewer deaths (12% vs 28%). Interestingly, those investigators did not see a clear difference in morbidity between anticoagulated (34%) and non-anticoagulated (40%) patients.[3] Southwick and colleagues[20] found that mortality decreased from 40% to 14%, and morbidity was decreased from 50% to 34% in patients who were anticoagulated. Levine and colleagues[32] found no significant decrease in mortality; however, those investigators did find a decrease in morbidity associated with anticoagulation. The proposed benefits of anticoagulation are the prevention of thrombus progression, inhibition of platelet function, antiinflammatory properties, and the promotion of antibiotic penetration in the thrombus.[3,5,7,32] Multiple anticoagulants have been used, including unfractionated heparin and low–molecular weight heparin, as well as multiple oral anticoagulants. No clear consensus on the treatment regimen exists; however, the authors recommend starting with rapidly reversible unfractionated heparin in initial stages of CST, followed by conversion to a long-acting agent when the patient's condition is stable, similar to that proposed by Bhatia and Jones.[17] Finally, the duration of anticoagulation is variable and should be continued until radiographic clearance of the CST is achieved; this generally ranges from several weeks to months.[5,7,17,28,29]

Surgical intervention is not a typical treatment for CST. In the case of a septic etiology, surgical intervention should be aimed at source control through surgical incision and drainage of any potential sources.[7] In the case of neoplastic CS syndrome leading to thrombosis, surgery may be beneficial in removing the offending mass lesion. When surgical intervention is performed, endoscopy is commonly employed to drain the sphenoid, ethmoidal, maxillary, and frontal sinuses.[3,5] Mastoidectomies and craniotomies (for empyema or abscess) may be performed along with orbital decompression, ventricular shunt placement (for post-infectious hydrocephalus), or both.[3,5]

SUMMARY

CST is a rare, but potentially lethal, condition that involves the formation of a thrombus resulting in venous hypertension within the CS secondary to either septic or aseptic etiologies. Aseptic etiologies include surgery, trauma, thrombophilia, neoplasia, head and neck cancers, hormone-replacement therapies, or pregnancy. Septic etiologies include sinusitis, otitis, erysipelas, mastoiditis, and odontogenic and facial infections. Evaluation of the patient begins with the clinical examination, which is important in identifying the many signs and symptoms that overlap with other, more common conditions.

It is imperative that clinicians maintain a reasonable degree of suspicion and move forward with appropriate imaging in the form of MR and CT modalities. Once a diagnosis or a high degree of suspicion is present, it is paramount to initiate appropriate therapies, which may include antibiotics, anticoagulants, and surgery for source control. Corticosteroids must be utilized judiciously because no clear consensus benefit has been established; however, they may be a necessity in patients with pituitary dysfunction or adrenal insufficiency.

CLINICS CARE POINTS

- CST is a rare and potentially lethal subset of cerebral sinus thrombosis that must be quickly identified and treated to produce the best possible outcome for the patient.
- CST has both septic and aseptic etiologies and affected patients may present with headache, "picket-fence" pyrexia, meningitic symptoms, facial hyperesthesia or hypoesthesia, chemosis, proptosis, ophthalmoplegia, vision loss, confusion, altered mentation, or even coma.
- Imaging modalities, such as 2-dimensional unenhanced time-of-flight and enhanced with elliptical centric view-ordering MR imaging and enhanced CT venography, are used to help establish the diagnosis when clinical suspicion exists.
- Treatments for CST mainly focus around the source and offending pathology control, which may include the need for antibiotics, anticoagulation, and surgery. Corticosteroid therapy is controversial but used in some cases based on clinician experience and preference.

ACKNOWLEDGMENTS

The authors thank Paul H. Dressel BFA for preparation of the illustrations and Carrie Owens MSILS and Debra J. Zimmer for editorial support.

DISCLOSURE

Dr J.M. Davies reports consulting fees, payment, or honoraria for lectures, presentations, speakers' bureaus, article writing, or educational events from Medtronic and Rapid Medical; support for attending meetings and/or travel from Medtronic and Rapid Medical; patents planned, issued, or pending from QAS.ai; participation on a data safety monitoring board or advisory board for the National Institutes of Health National Institute of Neurological Disorders and Stroke Strokenet; and stock or stock options from Synchron, Cerebrotech, and QAS.ai. No disclosures were reported by the other authors.

FUNDING

Research Grants: NIH R21/R01, NSF SBIR, UB-CAT, Buffalo Translational Consortium, Cummings Foundation, nVidia, Google. Financial Interest: QAS.ai, Rist Neurovascular, Cerebrotech, Synchron, HyperionConsultant/Advisory Board: Medtronic, Microvention, Imperative CareNational

PI/Steering Committees: StrokeNET DSMB, EMBOLISE, SUCCESS.

REFERENCES

1. Barranco-Trabi J, Scott JC, Fryer JM, et al. Unique presentation of septic cavernous sinus thrombosis and pulmonary embolism in the setting of reusable face covering. Case Rep Infect Dis 2022;2022:3388537.
2. McBane RD 2nd, Tafur A, Wysokinski WE. Acquired and congenital risk factors associated with cerebral venous sinus thrombosis. Thromb Res 2010;126(2): 81–7.
3. Weerasinghe D, Lueck CJ. Septic cavernous sinus thrombosis: case report and review of the literature. Neuro Ophthalmol 2016;40(6):263–76.
4. Qu H, Li Y, Chen M, et al. Cavernous sinus thrombosis: An insidious and dangerous "do-not-miss" diagnosis. Headache 2021;61(7):1144–9.
5. Caranfa JT, Yoon MK. Septic cavernous sinus thrombosis: A review. Surv Ophthalmol 2021;66(6):1021–30.
6. Idiculla PS, Gurala D, Palanisamy M, et al. Cerebral venous thrombosis: a comprehensive review. Eur Neurol 2020;83(4):369–79.
7. Desa V, Green R. Cavernous sinus thrombosis: current therapy. J Oral Maxillofac Surg 2012;70(9):2085–91.
8. Pannu AK, Saroch A, Sharma N. Danger triangle of face and septic cavernous sinus thrombosis. J Emerg Med 2017;53(1):137–8.
9. Lee JH, Lee HK, Park JK, et al. Cavernous sinus syndrome: clinical features and differential diagnosis with MR imaging. AJR Am J Roentgenol 2003;181(2):583–90.
10. Nambiar R, Nair SG. Cavernous sinus syndrome. SAVE Proc 2017;30(4):455–6.
11. Arimoto H, Shirotani T, Nakau H, et al. Primary malignant lymphoma of the cavernous sinus–case report. Neurol Med -Chir 2000;40(5):275–9.
12. Hirano H, Tashiro Y, Fujio S, et al. Diffuse large B-cell lymphoma within a cavernous hemangioma of the cavernous sinus. Brain Tumor Pathol 2011;28:353–8.
13. Huisman TA, Tschirch F, Schneider JF, et al. Burkitt's lymphoma with bilateral cavernous sinus and mediastinal involvement in a child. Pediatr Radiol 2003; 33(10):719–21.
14. Nakatomi H, Sasaki T, Kawamoto S, et al. Primary cavernous sinus malignant lymphoma treated by gamma knife radiosurgery: case report and review of the literature. Surg Neurol 1996;46(3):272–8. discussion 278-9.
15. de Bruijn SF, Stam J, Koopman MM, et al. Case-control study of risk of cerebral sinus thrombosis in oral contraceptive users and in [correction of who are] carriers of hereditary prothrombotic conditions. the cerebral venous sinus thrombosis study group. BMJ 1998;316(7131):589–92.
16. Plewa MC, Tadi P, Gupta M. Cavernous sinus thrombosis. StatPearls. StatPearls Publishing. July 31, 2023 (update). https://www.ncbi.nlm.nih.gov/books/NBK448177/. [Accessed 12 October 2023].
17. Bhatia K, Jones NS. Septic cavernous sinus thrombosis secondary to sinusitis: are anticoagulants indicated? A review of the literature. J Laryngol Otol 2002;116(9):667–76.
18. Colson AE, Daily JP. Orbital apex syndrome and cavernous sinus thrombosis due to infection with Staphylococcus aureus and Pseudomonas aeruginosa. Clin Infect Dis 1999;29(3):701–2.
19. DiNubile MJ. Septic thrombosis of the cavernous sinuses. Arch Neurol 1988;45(5):567–72.
20. Southwick FS, Richardson EP Jr, Swartz MN. Septic thrombosis of the dural venous sinuses. Medicine (Baltim) 1986;65(2):82–106.
21. Tveteras K, Kristensen S, Dommerby H. Septic cavernous and lateral sinus thrombosis: modern diagnostic and therapeutic principles. J Laryngol Otol 1988;102(10):877–82.
22. Shaw RE. Cavernous sinus thrombophlebitis: a review. Br J Surg 1952;40(159):40–8.
23. Leach JL, Fortuna RB, Jones BV, et al. Imaging of cerebral venous thrombosis: current techniques, spectrum of findings, and diagnostic pitfalls. Radiographics 2006;26(Suppl 1):S19–41. discussion S42-3.
24. Farb RI, Scott JN, Willinsky RA, et al. Intracranial venous system: gadolinium-enhanced three-dimensional MR venography with auto-triggered elliptic centric-ordered sequence–initial experience. Radiology 2003;226(1):203–9.
25. Wetzel SG, Kirsch E, Stock KW, et al. Cerebral veins: comparative study of CT venography with intraarterial digital subtraction angiography. AJNR Am J Neuroradiol 1999;20(2):249–55.
26. Ahmadi J, Keane JR, Segall HD, et al. CT observations pertinent to septic cavernous sinus thrombosis. AJNR Am J Neuroradiol 1985;6(5):755–8.
27. Bhatia H, Kaur R, Bedi R. MR imaging of cavernous sinus thrombosis. Eur J Radiol Open 2020;7:100226.
28. van der Poel NA, Mourits MP, de Win MML, et al. Prognosis of septic cavernous sinus thrombosis remarkably improved: a case series of 12 patients and literature review. Eur Arch Oto-Rhino-Laryngol 2018;275(9):2387–95.
29. Ebright JR, Pace MT, Niazi AF. Septic thrombosis of the cavernous sinuses. Arch Intern Med 2001; 161(22):2671–6.
30. Canhao P, Cortesao A, Cabral M, et al. Are steroids useful to treat cerebral venous thrombosis? Stroke 2008;39(1):105–10.
31. Khatri IA, Wasay M. Septic cerebral venous sinus thrombosis. J Neurol Sci 2016;362:221–7.
32. Levine SR, Twyman RE, Gilman S. The role of anticoagulation in cavernous sinus thrombosis. Neurology 1988;38(4):517.

Cerebrospinal Fluid-Venous Fistulas

Nitesh P. Patel, MD[a], Waleed Brinjikji, MD[a,b],*

KEYWORDS

- CSF-venous fistula • Spontaneous intracranial hypotension • CSF leak • Myelography
- Epidural blood patch • Transvenous embolization • Surgical nerve root ligation

KEY POINTS

- Cerebrospinal fluid-venous fistulas (CSFVFs) are being increasingly diagnosed as clinical and radiologic recognition improve.
- Lateral decubitus digital subtraction myelography is the current mainstay of CSFVF diagnosis.
- Epidural patching with autologous blood or fibrin glue typically only provides temporary symptomatic relief.
- Transvenous embolization is a minimally invasive treatment that provides durable symptomatic and radiographic improvement and will likely become the standard of care.
- Surgical ligation remains a durable treatment option but is more invasive and is limited at eloquent levels, including the cervical and lumbar regions.

INTRODUCTION

Spontaneous intracranial hypotension (SIH) results from 1 of 3 types of spinal cerebrospinal fluid (CSF) leaks: a linear dural tear either ventral or posterolateral to the spinal cord, leakage from a meningeal diverticulum, or a spinal CSF-venous fistula (CSFVF).[1] Since first described in a series of 3 cases by Schievink and colleagues[2] in 2014, CSFVFs have become an increasingly recognized cause of SIH. Although the exact pathogenesis has yet to be defined, aberrant fistulous connections between the spinal CSF space and adjacent paraspinal veins allow for unregulated loss of CSF into venous system, thereby resulting in CSF depletion and the eventual clinical and radiologic manifestations of intracranial hypotension. In this review, we discuss the epidemiology and clinical presentation of CSFVF, provide a simple diagnostic paradigm with a summary of recent advancements in diagnostic imaging techniques, and present appropriate treatment strategies. Finally, we will briefly discuss avenues of future research.

EPIDEMIOLOGY

The annual incidence of SIH is estimated at approximately 4 per 100,000 population.[3,4] In 2016, Schievink and colleagues[1] published a classification system for spontaneous spinal CSF leaks and found that CSFVF, classified as a type 3 CSF leak, only accounted for 2.5% of the 568 patients who presented to their institution with SIH from 2009 to 2015. At that time, CSFVF was a newly recognized cause of spontaneous spinal CSF leaks and only a few cases had been reported in the literature. Advancements in diagnostic methods, particularly lateral decubitus digital subtraction myelography (LDDSM), along with growing clinical recognition of the condition, have led to increased CSFVF diagnosis over recent years, indicating that the condition accounts for a greater fraction of SIH cases than initially expected. While larger scale epidemiologic studies are not available, CSFVF accounted for 50% of patients presenting with SIH in our recent population-based study of SIH in Olmsted County.[3] We suspect that the overall prevalence

a Department of Neurosurgery, Mayo Clinic, 200 1st Street Southwest, Rochester, MN 55905, USA;
b Department of Radiology, Mayo Clinic, 200 1st Street Southwest, Rochester, MN 55905, USA
* Corresponding author. 200 1st Street Southwest, Rochester, MN 55905.
E-mail address: Brinjikji.Waleed@mayo.edu

Neurosurg Clin N Am 35 (2024) 311–318
https://doi.org/10.1016/j.nec.2024.02.003

of CSFVF is likely underestimated and the incidence will continue to increase as clinical recognition increases, diagnostic methods become more widely available, and optimal diagnostic techniques and modalities are discovered.

In our experience, women are more commonly affected by CSFVF than men, with a female/male ratio of approximately 2:1. The patient population is mostly middle-aged adults (40–60 years) who are otherwise generally healthy without major medical comorbidities. Most CSFVFs are found in the thoracic spine, particularly in the right T5 to T12 region; however, published cases series have presented conflicting data on laterality predominance.[5–13] Cervical, lumbar, and sacral CSFVFs have been observed, but they are less common compared to the thoracic region.[10,14,15]

CLINICAL PRESENTATION

CSFVFs present with symptoms of SIH, of which the cardinal symptom is orthostatic headache, a type of headache that worsens when upright and improves with recumbency. Some patients report headache onset instantaneously after assuming an upright position, whereas others report headache development minutes to hours after being upright.[16] In a much smaller subset of patients, there is a several-hour delay of onset that occurs during the afternoon hours, which has been termed "second-half-of-the-day" headache.[17] Prior efforts aimed at understanding the natural history of SIH showed that the orthostatic component of the headache can diminish over time.[18] Although orthostatic headache is the most common headache type, other patterns have been reported, including Valsalva-induced, exertional, thunderclap, and even reverse orthostatic.[19–21] Notably, Valsalva-induced headache worsening appears to be more common in patients with CSFVFs.[6] The range of headache patterns can lead to delays in diagnosis, especially in the subset of patients in which headache is not present at all.

Additional clinical manifestations include a myriad of nonspecific symptoms that add further challenge to arriving at an accurate diagnosis. Many patients report "brain fog," described as difficulty with concentration and word finding.[6] A smaller number of patients present with striking early-onset dementia similar to behavioral-variant frontotemporal dementia, likely from downward sagging of the frontal and temporal lobes secondary to CSF depletion. These patients exhibit disinhibited behavior, executive dysfunction, and personality changes.[22] Aural symptoms are reported in about one-third of patients and include hearing loss, muffled hearing, phonophobia, and pulsatile tinnitus. Visual symptoms, such as photophobia, blurred vision, and diplopia, occur less frequently. Movement disorders including tremor, choreiform movements, parkinsonism, and gait ataxia have been observed. Other symptoms include posterior neck pain or stiffness, nausea, vomiting, and vertigo.[6,16,17,23,24] In rare cases, severe brain sag can result in diencephalic brainstem compression and subsequent coma.[25]

DIAGNOSIS

Per the International Classification of Headache Disorders, third edition, the diagnostic criteria of SIH include either low CSF pressure (<6 cm CSF) or imaging evidence of CSF leak, headache that developed in temporal relation to the low CSF pressure or leakage of CSF, or any headache that is not better accounted for by a different diagnosis.[26] Despite these criteria, low opening pressure has only been reported in up to one-third of patients with confirmed SIH and is therefore an unreliable diagnostic marker. Instead, patients presenting with clinical manifestations of SIH should undergo a careful, stepwise imaging evaluation of the brain and spine. Practitioners evaluating patients with SIH should be aware of the imaging modalities employed in order to identify the CSF leak, especially in cases of CSFVF, given that precise localization is imperative for guiding targeted treatment and maximizing treatment outcome.

Cranial Imaging Findings in Spontaneous Intracranial Hypotension

Features of SIH on brain MRI can be remembered by the mnemonic SEEPS: subdural fluid collections, enhancement of the pachymeninges, engorgement of venous structures, pituitary hyperemia, and sagging of the brain. A validated scoring system developed by Dobrocky and colleagues[27] assigns point values to the most common brain MRI findings of SIH and can predict the likelihood (low, intermediate, high) of diagnosing an underlying CSF leak on subsequent myelography based on the cumulative score, referred to as the Bern SIH score. However, it is important to note that cranial imaging can be normal in approximately 20% of patients with SIH.[28]

Evolution of Diagnostic Methods for Cerebrospinal Fluid-Venous Fistulas

The first 3 cases of CSFVFs reported in the literature were identified on prone digital subtraction myelography (DSM). DSM allows for real-time high spatial and temporal resolution imaging of contrast injected into the thecal sac via lumbar puncture and is therefore a valuable method for diagnosing spontaneous CSF leak.[29] Performing DSM in the prone position causes maximal contrast pooling in the ventral aspect of the thecal sac due to gravity, which makes this technique an excellent choice for localizing a CSF leak secondary to a ventral dural tear. However, since CSFVFs are located laterally along the thecal sac or along a nerve root sleeve, there is lack of sufficient contrast in the lateral gutters on prone DSM to opacify the fistulous vein(s). This results in a detection rate as low as 19% in 1 study.[8]

Performing DSM in the lateral decubitus position allows increased contrast concentration in the lateral (dependent) part of the thecal sac and thereby maximizes the amount of contrast near the fistulous connection, which in turn dramatically increases the diagnostic yield to 70%.[7] The improved detection rate of LDDSM was corroborated in a study that showed a nearly 5-fold increase in CSFVF detection (diagnostic yield of 74%) versus DSM in the prone position (diagnostic yield of 15%).[30]

CSFVFs are challenging to detect since many of them opacify only intermittently following intrathecal contrast injection. While LDDSM is the mainstay of CSFVF localization in our practice due to its superior temporal and spatial resolution, DSM is not widely available and requires radiologists who are familiar with interventional techniques. Lateral decubitus computed tomography myelography (LDCTM) is a more widely available diagnostic method that has reasonable diagnostic yield for CSFVFs, and bilateral LDCTM can be performed safely in a single session rather than over separate days.[5,9,31] The "hyperdense paraspinal vein" sign on computed tomography (CT) myelography has shown to correlate with the level and laterality of a paravertebral or lateral CSFVF.[32] However, this sign may not be present in cases of CSFVFs that drain centrally into the internal vertebral venous plexus; in these cases, the "hyperdense basivertebral vein" sign has been proposed as a CT marker for central drainage of a CSFVF.[33]

Diagnostic Workflow for Cerebrospinal Fluid Leaks at Mayo Clinic

Patients presenting to our institution with clinical suspicion of SIH are evaluated in our CSF dynamics clinic by neurologists with subspecialty focus in headache and intracranial hypotension. The initial workup includes MRI of the brain and entire spine. Brain MRI is used to evaluate for the aforementioned features of SIH, which can be scored using the Bern SIH scoring system to predict the pretest probability of subsequent spinal myelography. Patients with higher Bern SIH score have a higher likelihood of CSF leak discovery on subsequent myelography, and patients with a Bern SIH score ≤2 can likely forego myelography unless there is a high clinical suspicion of SIH.[11] Spine MRI is used to evaluate for a spinal longitudinal extradural collection (SLEC), which if present indicates an underlying fast CSF leak from a ventral or posterolateral dural tear; in this situation, the patient proceeds to prone dynamic CT myelogram to localize the dural tear and guide targeted treatment.[34]

CSF leaks directly into the venous system in patients with CSFVF, so these patients will not have an SLEC identified on spine MRI. For patients with a high clinical suspicion of SIH with or without associated brain MRI findings and no presence of SLEC on spine MRI, the evaluation proceeds directly to LDDSM. We typically perform LDDSM on 2 consecutive days with subsequent dual-energy same-side decubitus CT myelography on each day, starting with the patient in the right lateral decubitus position on day 1.[35] Regardless of whether a leak is identified on day 1, we proceed with the left lateral decubitus position on day 2 given that a small percentage of patients have bilateral leaks.[11] Importantly, we have not observed any major adverse effects after performing LDDSM on 2 consecutive days.[36]

Recent Advancements in Diagnostic Modalities

Despite the high spatial and temporal resolution of LDDSM, up to one-third of patients with high probability Bern SIH score (>5) may not have a CSF leak identified.[11] Thus, continued investigation of the optimal imaging method is necessary to appropriately diagnose and care for patients with a suspected CSFVF. One approach is to perform same-side LDCTM approximately 10 to 30 minutes after a negative LDDSM, which has shown to provide an incremental diagnostic yield up to 38.6%.[37] Even if a CSFVF is not explicitly identified on the LDCTM, the laterality of a CSFVF can be indirectly inferred by evaluating the degree of renal contrast accumulation.[38,39] Specifically, there is greater accumulation of renal contrast on LDCTM following LDDSM when the patient is lying in the decubitus position ipsilateral to a CSFVF. By learning the laterality of the CSFVF, future repeat LDDSM can be focused on the side of interest. Cone beam CT (CBCT) is another adjunct in patients who have indeterminate LDDSM findings by providing 3-dimensional visualization of the potential areas of interest. In our recent study, we showed that in 15 patients with indeterminate LDDSM findings, subsequent CBCT detected a CSFVF in 7 patients.[13]

Photon-counting detector CT myelography (PCDCTM) performed in the lateral decubitus position is an exciting new technology that has shown great promise for detecting CSFVF. The first report of a CSFVF diagnosed with PCDCTM showed a much clearer depiction of the fistulous draining veins.[40] This is due to the high temporal resolution, exquisite spatial resolution, and spectral imaging capabilities of PCDCTM, which make the technology theoretically more sensitive for detecting CSFVFs. In the 6 patients diagnosed with a CSFVF using PCDCTM in our small series, 3 patients had an initial negative LDDSM and 2 patients had prior negative LDCTM. An example of a right T8 CSFVF diagnosed on PCDCTM in a patient with negative LDDSM is shown in **Fig. 1**. While accessibility to PCDCTM is not widespread at this time, the imaging modality is an excellent way to investigate for a CSFVF in patients in whom there is a high clinical suspicion but prior LDDSM or LDCTM was negative. Ultimately, PCDCTM may become the initial myelographic test of choice to localize CSFVF as it becomes more widely available.[41]

TREATMENT

Three main treatment options have emerged for patients with CSFVF: (1) percutaneous epidural patching, either using autologous blood (commonly known as a "blood patch") or fibrin glue; (2) transvenous embolization using a liquid embolic agent; and (3) open surgical intervention. There are no randomized data comparing these treatments; however, transvenous embolization and open surgery have shown the most durable outcomes. We will briefly discuss all 3 treatment options.

Epidural Patching with Autologous Blood or Fibrin Glue

Percutaneous epidural patching has been the historical standard of care for patients with a spontaneous CSF leak and is theorized to provide benefit by compressing the area of leakage. In our experience, epidural patching provides temporary symptomatic improvement but is typically unsuccessful in providing durable symptomatic relief in patients with CSFVF compared to other types of CSF leak. This appears consistent with findings from other studies.[5–7,17,32]

More recently, Mamlouk and colleagues[42] reported encouraging results of CT-guided fibrin glue occlusion of CSFVFs. In their initial retrospective case series, all 13 patients had complete symptomatic resolution as well as radiologic improvement on posttreatment brain MRI; however, the follow-up period was short for most patients. Their subsequent study included 35 patients with longer follow-up and showed that CT-guided fibrin glue occlusion of CSFVFs provided durable symptomatic and radiologic improvement.[43]

Transvenous Embolization

In 2021, we presented our novel endovascular transvenous CSFVF embolization technique in a series of the first 5 patients treated with this method.[44] We refer the reader to the previously published technical report or our technical video

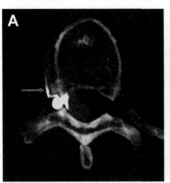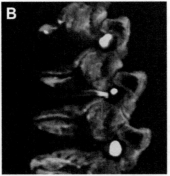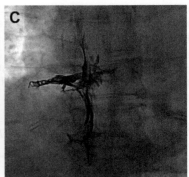

Fig. 1. Example of a right T8 cerebrospinal fluid-venous fistula (CSFVF) on photon counting detector computed tomography myelography (*A*) Axial image at the T8 spinal level demonstrating a nerve root sleeve diverticulum with opacification of the right T8 paraspinal vein (*red arrow*), indicative of a right T8 CSFVF. (*B*) Sagittal image demonstrating opacification of the right T8 paraspinal vein (*red arrow*). (*C*) Fluoroscopic image following successful transvenous Onyx embolization of the right T8 CSFVF; the Onyx cast involves the paraspinal vein, intercostal vein, foraminal veins, and epidural venous plexus.

for procedural details.[44,45] The goal of the procedure is to prevent CSF leakage into the venous system by using Onyx, a liquid embolic agent, to endovascularly embolize the intercostal vein, paraspinal vein, foraminal vein, and internal epidural venous plexus at the spinal level and side of the patient's CSFVF. This results in either direct occlusion of the fistula by the liquid embolic agent or local venous hypertension that reverses the favorable pressure gradient that initially allowed CSF leakage through the fistulous connection into the vein.

Our subsequent report of clinical and radiologic outcomes of 40 patients who underwent this therapy showed positive results on short-term follow-up: 83% of patients had much improved or very much improved Patient Global Impression of Change (PGIC), there was a large statistically significant reduction in Headache Impact Test (HIT-6) scores, and greater than 90% of patients had concordant radiologic improvement on brain MRI as measured by Bern SIH score.[10] Parizadeh and colleagues[46] reported similar clinical and radiographic improvement in 18 patients who underwent transvenous CSFVF embolization at their institution. The short follow-up period for each of these studies precludes definitive conclusions regarding the durability of the treatment method; however, we have observed long-lasting therapeutic effects over time and results of long-term follow-up are forthcoming. We hypothesize that fistula recanalization is unlikely given that Onyx is a permanent embolic agent and CSFVF are slow-flow shunts with small pressure gradients.

Smaller cases series of transvenous embolization have been published from other institutions, including a community-based academic hospital in California and a hospital in Italy.[47,48] Both showed clinical and radiographic improvement on short-term follow-up and demonstrate that the treatment method can be reproduced outside of major academic referral centers. Given the effectiveness and minimally invasive nature of the procedure, we believe that transvenous embolization will likely become the first-line treatment option for patients with CSFVFs and will be of particular importance in patients with multiple fistulas or a fistula at an eloquent spinal level.

Surgery

Prior to the introduction of transvenous embolization, laminectomy or hemilaminectomy with partial or complete facetectomy was the mainstay of accessing and definitively treating CSFVFs.[2,5,6,8,49,50] Exposure of the lateral thecal sac and nerve root sleeve at the level of the CSFVF allows for direct visualization of the dilated fistula vein(s). Aside for the T1 level, the nerve roots in the thoracic spine can sacrificed by ligating adjacent to the thecal sac and proximal to the dorsal root ganglion, which will obliterate the fistula; care must be taken to ensure the artery of Adamkiewicz or a large radiculomedullary artery is not associated with the nerve root prior to surgery. All other levels of the spine are eloquent levels where the nerve root cannot be sacrificed, in which case the vein(s) are stripped from the nerve root and coagulated with bipolar cautery.[15]

Positive clinical outcomes have been reported following surgical treatment of CSFVFs. In our recent retrospective review of 25 patients undergoing surgical treatment for CSFVFs, 92% of patients with headaches reported partial or complete headache improvement postoperatively, though improvement in associated Bern score varied from no improvement to complete improvement.[15] The only prospective study of clinical outcomes following surgical ligation of CSFVF revealed significant improvement in HIT-6 scores in the 20 patients that were included in the study, and all patients reported high level of satisfaction on the PGIC questionnaire.[50]

Schievink and colleagues[51] showed that surgical ligation is feasible and effective in patients who have previously failed transvenous embolization. In their small series of 6 patients, the Onyx-containing veins were found to be compressible and easily resectable, which facilitated surgical occlusion of the fistula. Complete symptom resolution was achieved in 5 of the 6 patients, and all patients had radiologic resolution of brain MRI findings. Recently, the use of intraoperative intrathecal fluorescein allowed for visualization of a residual CSFVF following prior incomplete Onyx embolization.[52]

The first report of a minimally invasive surgical approach to CSFVF ligation showed successful outcomes in a recent series of 5 patients.[53] Mini-laminectomy and foraminotomy were performed via a percutaneous minimally invasive tubular retractor system. This provided visualization of the lateral thecal sac, exiting nerve root, and the CSFVF, which was ligated successfully in all patients without complication. All patients had clinical and radiographic improvement at the 6-month follow-up.

Ultimately, surgical intervention, either via traditional open surgery or a minimally invasive approach, remains a definitive treatment option for patients with CSFVFs.

CHALLENGES AND FUTURE DIRECTIONS

We have gained significant knowledge regarding the epidemiology, presentation, diagnosis, and treatment of CSFVF since the pathology was first described nearly a decade ago. Despite this, many questions remain, including etiopathogenesis, optimal diagnostic modality, and standard of care treatment. Several clinical challenges also need to be addressed, including rebound hypertension following fistula treatment, management of patients with multiple CSFVFs, and modes of further investigation in patients with a high clinical suspicion for CSFVF but negative imaging studies.

CLINICS CARE POINTS

- Cerebrospinal fluid-venous fistulas (CSFVFs) are an increasingly recognized cause of spontaneous intracranial hypotension.
- Lateral decubitus digital subtraction myelography is the current mainstay of CSFVF diagnosis.
- Epidural patching with autologous blood or fibrin glue typically only provides temporary symptomatic relief.
- Transvenous embolization is a minimally invasive treatment that provides durable symptomatic and radiographic improvement and will likely become the standard of care.
- Surgical ligation remains a durable treatment option but is more invasive and is limited at eloquent levels, including the cervical and lumbar regions.

DISCLOSURE

The authors have nothing to disclose.

REFERENCES

1. Schievink WI, Maya MM, Jean-Pierre S, et al. A classification system of spontaneous spinal CSF leaks. Neurology 2016;87(7):673–9.
2. Schievink WI, Moser FG, Maya MM. CSF-venous fistula in spontaneous intracranial hypotension. Neurology 2014;83(5):472–3.
3. Pradeep A, Madhavan AA, Brinjikji W, et al. Incidence of spontaneous intracranial hypotension in Olmsted County, Minnesota: 2019-2021. Interv Neuroradiol 2023. 15910199231165429.
4. Schievink WI, Maya MM, Moser FG, et al. Incidence of spontaneous intracranial hypotension in a community: Beverly Hills, California, 2006-2020. Cephalalgia 2022;42(4–5):312–6.
5. Kranz PG, Amrhein TJ, Gray L. CSF Venous Fistulas in Spontaneous Intracranial Hypotension: Imaging Characteristics on Dynamic and CT Myelography. AJR Am J Roentgenol 2017;209(6):1360–6.
6. Duvall JR, Robertson CE, Cutsforth-Gregory JK, et al. Headache due to spontaneous spinal cerebrospinal fluid leak secondary to cerebrospinal fluid-venous fistula: Case series. Cephalalgia 2019;39(14):1847–54.
7. Farb RI, Nicholson PJ, Peng PW, et al. Spontaneous Intracranial Hypotension: A Systematic Imaging Approach for CSF Leak Localization and Management Based on MRI and Digital Subtraction Myelography. AJNR Am J Neuroradiol 2019;40(4):745–53.
8. Schievink WI, Moser FG, Maya MM, et al. Digital subtraction myelography for the identification of spontaneous spinal CSF-venous fistulas. J Neurosurg Spine 2016;24(6):960–4.
9. Mamlouk MD, Ochi RP, Jun P, et al. Decubitus CT Myelography for CSF-Venous Fistulas: A Procedural Approach. AJNR Am J Neuroradiol 2021;42(1):32–6.
10. Brinjikji W, Garza I, Whealy M, et al. Clinical and imaging outcomes of cerebrospinal fluid-venous fistula embolization. J Neurointerventional Surg 2022;14(10):953–6.
11. Kim DK, Carr CM, Benson JC, et al. Diagnostic Yield of Lateral Decubitus Digital Subtraction Myelogram Stratified by Brain MRI Findings. Neurology 2021;96(9):e1312–8.
12. Borg N, Cutsforth-Gregory J, Oushy S, et al. Anatomy of Spinal Venous Drainage for the Neurointerventionalist: From Puncture Site to Intervertebral Foramen. AJNR Am J Neuroradiol 2022;43(4):517–25.
13. Madhavan AA, Cutsforth-Gregory JK, Benson JC, et al. Conebeam CT as an Adjunct to Digital Subtraction Myelography for Detection of CSF-Venous Fistulas. AJNR Am J Neuroradiol 2023;44(3):347–50.
14. Mark IT, Morris PP, Brinjikji W, et al. Sacral CSF-Venous Fistulas and Potential Imaging Techniques. AJNR Am J Neuroradiol 2022;43(12):1824–6.
15. Montenegro MM, Kissoon NR, Atkinson JLD, et al. Clinical and Imaging Outcomes of Surgically Repaired Cerebrospinal Fluid-Venous Fistulas Identified by Lateral Decubitus Digital Subtraction Myelography. World Neurosurg 2023. https://doi.org/10.1016/j.wneu.2023.06.062.
16. Schievink WI. Spontaneous Intracranial Hypotension. N Engl J Med 2021;385(23):2173–8.
17. Shlobin NA, Shah VN, Chin CT, et al. Cerebrospinal Fluid-Venous Fistulas: A Systematic Review and Examination of Individual Patient Data. Neurosurgery 2021;88(5):931–41.
18. Häni L, Fung C, Jesse CM, et al. Insights into the natural history of spontaneous intracranial hypotension from infusion testing. Neurology 2020;95(3):e247–55.
19. Mokri B, Aksamit AJ, Atkinson JLD. Paradoxical postural headaches in cerebrospinal fluid leaks. Cephalalgia 2004;24(10):883–7.

20. Mokri B, Posner JB. Spontaneous intracranial hypotension: the broadening clinical and imaging spectrum of CSF leaks. Neurology 2000;55(12):1771–2.

21. Chang T, Rodrigo C, Samarakoon L. Spontaneous intracranial hypotension presenting as thunderclap headache: a case report. BMC Res Notes 2015;8:108.

22. Schievink WI, Maya M, Barnard Z, et al. The reversible impairment of behavioral variant frontotemporal brain sagging syndrome: Challenges and opportunities. Alzheimers Dement 2022;8(1):e12367.

23. Roytman M, Salama G, Robbins MS, et al. CSF-Venous Fistula. Curr Pain Headache Rep 2021;25(1):5.

24. Kumar R, Cutsforth-Gregory JK, Brinjikji W. Cerebrospinal Fluid Leaks, Spontaneous Intracranial Hypotension, and Chiari I Malformation. Neurosurg Clin 2023;34(1):185–92.

25. Carlstrom LP, Oushy S, Graffeo CS, et al. Intracranial Hypotensive Crisis From an Insidious Spinal Cerebrospinal Fluid-Venous Fistula: A Case Report. Oper Neurosurg (Hagerstown) 2021;21(3):E283–8.

26. Headache Classification Committee of the International Headache Society (IHS). The International Classification of Headache Disorders, 3rd edition (beta version). Cephalalgia 2013;33(9):629–808.

27. Dobrocky T, Grunder L, Breiding PS, et al. Assessing Spinal Cerebrospinal Fluid Leaks in Spontaneous Intracranial Hypotension With a Scoring System Based on Brain Magnetic Resonance Imaging Findings. JAMA Neurol 2019;76(5):580–7.

28. Schievink WI. Spontaneous spinal cerebrospinal fluid leaks and intracranial hypotension. JAMA 2006;295(19):2286–96.

29. Hoxworth JM, Trentman TL, Kotsenas AL, et al. The role of digital subtraction myelography in the diagnosis and localization of spontaneous spinal CSF leaks. AJR Am J Roentgenol 2012;199(3):649–53.

30. Schievink WI, Maya MM, Moser FG, et al. Lateral decubitus digital subtraction myelography to identify spinal CSF-venous fistulas in spontaneous intracranial hypotension. J Neurosurg Spine 2019;31(6):1–4.

31. Carlton Jones L, Goadsby PJ. Same-Day Bilateral Decubitus CT Myelography for Detecting CSF-Venous Fistulas in Spontaneous Intracranial Hypotension. AJNR Am J Neuroradiol 2022;43(4):645–8.

32. Kranz PG, Amrhein TJ, Schievink WI, et al. The "hyperdense paraspinal vein" sign: a marker of csf-venous fistula. AJNR Am J Neuroradiol 2016;37(7):1379–81.

33. Lützen N, Kremers N, Fung C, et al. The "hyperdense basivertebral vein" sign: another marker of a CSF-venous fistula. Neuroradiology 2022;64(3):627–30.

34. Luetmer PH, Schwartz KM, Eckel LJ, et al. When should I do dynamic CT myelography? Predicting fast spinal CSF leaks in patients with spontaneous intracranial hypotension. AJNR Am J Neuroradiol 2012;33(4):690–4.

35. Kim DK, Brinjikji W, Morris PP, et al. Lateral Decubitus Digital Subtraction Myelography: Tips, Tricks, and Pitfalls. AJNR Am J Neuroradiol 2020;41(1):21–8.

36. Pope MC, Carr CM, Brinjikji W, et al. Safety of Consecutive Bilateral Decubitus Digital Subtraction Myelography in Patients with Spontaneous Intracranial Hypotension and Occult CSF Leak. AJNR Am J Neuroradiol 2020;41(10):1953–7.

37. Shlapak DP, Mark IT, Kim DK, et al. Incremental diagnostic yield and clinical outcomes of lateral decubitus CT myelogram immediately following negative lateral decubitus digital subtraction myelogram. Neuroradiol J 2023;36(5):593–600.

38. Farb RI, O'Reilly ST, Hendriks EJ, et al. Spontaneous intracranial hypotension due to CSF-venous fistula: Evaluation of renal accumulation of contrast following decubitus myelography and maintained decubitus CT to improve fistula localization. Interv Neuroradiol 2023. 15910199231172627.

39. Wagle S, Benson JC, Madhavan AA, et al. The clue is in the kidneys: greater renal contrast medium accumulation on ipsilateral side down CT myelogram after lateral decubitus digital subtraction myelogram as a predictor of laterality of cerebrospinal fluid leak. Clin Radiol 2023;78(9):e608–12.

40. Schwartz FR, Malinzak MD, Amrhein TJ. Photon-Counting Computed Tomography Scan of a Cerebrospinal Fluid Venous Fistula. JAMA Neurol 2022;79(6):628–9.

41. Madhavan AA, Yu L, Brinjikji W, et al. Utility of Photon-Counting Detector CT Myelography for the Detection of CSF-Venous Fistulas. AJNR Am J Neuroradiol 2023;44(6):740–4.

42. Mamlouk MD, Shen PY, Sedrak MF, et al. CT-guided Fibrin Glue Occlusion of Cerebrospinal Fluid-Venous Fistulas. Radiology 2021;299(2):409–18.

43. Mamlouk MD, Shen PY, Dahlin BC. Headache response after CT-guided fibrin glue occlusion of CSF-venous fistulas. Headache 2022;62(8):1007–18.

44. Brinjikji W, Savastano LE, Atkinson JLD, et al. A Novel Endovascular Therapy for CSF Hypotension Secondary to CSF-Venous Fistulas. AJNR Am J Neuroradiol 2021;42(5):882–7.

45. Borg N, Oushy S, Savastano L, et al. Transvenous embolization of a cerebrospinal fluid-venous fistula for the treatment of spontaneous intracranial hypotension. J Neurointerventional Surg 2022;14(9):948.

46. Parizadeh D, Fermo O, Vibhute P, et al. Transvenous embolization of cerebrospinal fluid-venous fistulas: Independent validation and feasibility of upper-extremity approach and using dual-microcatheter and balloon pressure cooker

technique. J Neurointerv Surg 2023. https://doi.org/10.1136/jnis-2022-019946.

47. Noufal M, Liang CW, Negus J. Transvenous Embolization for Cerebrospinal Fluid-Venous Fistula. A Case Series from a Single Community-Academic Center. World Neurosurg 2022;168:e613–20.

48. Bergui M, Mistretta F, Bosco G, et al. CSF-venous leak responsible for spontaneous intracranial hypotension treated by endovascular venous route: First cases in Italy. Interv Neuroradiol 2022. 15910199221116011.

49. Kumar N, Diehn FE, Carr CM, et al. Spinal CSF venous fistula: A treatable etiology for CSF leaks in craniospinal hypovolemia. Neurology 2016;86(24):2310–2.

50. Wang TY, Karikari IO, Amrhein TJ, et al. Clinical Outcomes Following Surgical Ligation of Cerebrospinal Fluid-Venous Fistula in Patients With Spontaneous Intracranial Hypotension: A Prospective Case Series. Oper Neurosurg (Hagerstown) 2020;18(3):239–45.

51. Schievink WI, Tache RB, Maya MM. Surgical Ligation of Spinal CSF-Venous Fistulas after Transvenous Embolization in Patients with Spontaneous Intracranial Hypotension. AJNR Am J Neuroradiol 2022;43(7):1073–6.

52. Häni L, El Rahal A, Fung C, et al. Intraoperative Visualization of Flow in Direct Cerebrospinal Fluid-Venous Fistulas Using Intrathecal Fluorescein. Oper Neurosurg (Hagerstown). 2023;24(5):e336–41.

53. Lohkamp LN, Marathe N, Nicholson P, et al. Minimally invasive surgery for spinal cerebrospinal fluid-venous fistula ligation: patient series. J Neurosurg Case Lessons 2022;3(18). https://doi.org/10.3171/CASE21730.

Carotid Cavernous Fistula

Brian M. Howard, MD[a,b,]*, Daniel L. Barrow, MD[a]

KEYWORDS

- Cavernous sinus • Fistula • Dural • Arteriovenous fistula • Carotid artery

KEY POINTS

- Carotid cavernous fistulae (CCFs) are arteriovenous shunting lesions involving the cavernous sinus and are defined as direct or indirect.
- Direct CCFs are treated with either internal carotid artery deconstruction or reconstruction depending on the clinical scenario.
- Indirect CCFs are treated as dural fistulae of the cavernous sinus, most commonly, via transvenous, endovascular techniques.

INTRODUCTION

Carotid cavernous fistulae (CCF) are arteriovenous shunting lesions in which the cavernous sinus is pressurized by arterial blood. CCFs are historically characterized as direct when they arise from the internal carotid artery (ICA) proper, most commonly via a ruptured cavernous segment aneurysm, or from traumatic ICA injury or indirect, in which the arterial supply is via dural branches of the cavernous sinus from the ICA and/or external carotid artery (ECA).[1] Commonly referred to as "pulsating exophthalmos"—a common presenting symptom—throughout the nineteenth and much of the early twentieth century, the first report of a direct CCF dates to 1811, when Benjamin Travers published his account of treating a 34-year-old woman with a ruptured cavernous segment ICA aneurysm by ligature of the common carotid artery in 1804 at Guy's Hospital.[2] The first description of an indirect CCF is from 1864, in which Aubry of Rennes describes having treated what he believed to be a direct CCF 9 years previously, but on dissection of the cavernous sinus after arterial injection at autopsy was assuredly what is now recognized as an indirect CCF.[3,4] The authors' understanding of the pathology, workup, and treatment of CCFs has advanced dramatically over

the nearly 220 years since their first description and will be the focus of this review.

NATURE OF THE PROBLEM: ANATOMY

The cavernous sinus is a complex anatomic structure in the parasellar region at the confluence of the anterior and central skull base. At the most basic level, the cavernous sinuses are paired dural envelopes flanking either side of the sella, pituitary gland, and sphenoid sinus.[5] In addition to venous blood, the cavernous sinus contains the cavernous segment of the ICA and multiple cranial nerves, including the oculomotor, trochlear, abducens, and the ophthalmic (V1) and maxillary (V2) components of the trigeminal. As a chamber containing venous blood, the cavernous sinus receives input from the superior and inferior ophthalmic veins, Sylvian veins, and veins associated with the anterior and middle fossae and communicates with surrounding dural venous sinuses, such as the basilar or clival sinus, the inferior and superior petrosal sinuses, and the sphenoparietal sinus, as well as the pterygoid plexus.[5] Each cavernous sinus is interconnected via the inferior and superior intercavernous sinuses. In the setting of direct CCF, the arterial anatomy of relevance is the cavernous segment of the ICA proper. Dural blood vessels

[a] Department of Neurosurgery, Emory University School of Medicine, 1365 Clifton Road Northeast, Suite. B6200, Atlanta, GE 30322, USA; [b] Department of Radiology and Imaging Sciences, Division of Interventional Neuroradiology, Emory University School of Medicine, 1364 Clifton Road NE, AG26, Atlanta, GE 30322, USA
* Corresponding author. Department of Neurosurgery, Emory University School of Medicine, 1365 Clifton Road Northeast, Suite. B6200, Atlanta, GE 30322.
E-mail address: brian.howard@emory.edu

Neurosurg Clin N Am 35 (2024) 319–329
https://doi.org/10.1016/j.nec.2024.02.004
1042-3680/24/© 2024 Elsevier Inc. All rights reserved.

that commonly supply indirect CCF include branches of the meningohypophyseal and inferolateral trunks from the ICA and the middle meningeal artery, ascending pharyngeal artery, and the artery of foramen rotundum from the ECA. Thorough understanding of cavernous sinus anatomy is critical to evaluate clinical syndromes by which CCFs present and in deciding which treatment paradigm is likely to maximize the potential for cure while minimizing the likelihood of complications.

NATURE OF THE PROBLEM: PATHOPHYSIOLOGY

The most common pathophysiologic mechanisms of direct CCFs are rupture of a cavernous segment ICA aneurysm or trauma. Mechanisms of traumatic, direct CCF include penetrating trauma with laceration of the carotid artery or blunt trauma with either dissection sufficient to result in a tear through all three arterial layers or transection. The cavernous segment of the ICA is prone to injury in the setting of blunt trauma, either by direct injury in the setting of skull base fracture or due to shear force applied to the cavernous ICA—which is mobile but between the fixed petrous and clinoidal segments.[6–8] Iatrogenic injury of the cavernous segment of the ICA can occur in a variety of procedures, which is quite rare, but is most common during endoscopic, endonasal skull base surgery with a frequency of around 0.25% to 0.5%.[9,10]

Indirect CCFs are essentially dural arteriovenous fistulae (dAVF) of the cavernous sinus. The pathogenesis of dAVF remains unclear; however, human observational studies and animal models indicate that dural venous sinus or cortical vein thrombosis may lead to a proangiogenic milieu that results in aberrant arteriovenous shunting within the dura.[11–13] Indirect evidence supporting this hypothesis is the increased occurrence of various genes associated with hypercoagulable states in patients who harbor a dAVF.[14] Both clinical and experimental data suggest that venous hypertension alone is sufficient to upregulate proangiogenic factors such as basic fibroblast growth factor, and others, and cause formation of dAVF.[13,15]

NATURE OF THE PROBLEM: CLASSIFICATION

The Barrow classification is the most commonly used system to stratify CCFs.[1] Type A fistulae are characterized as a direct, high-flow shunt between the ICA and cavernous sinus. Types B to D are variations of dAVF of the cavernous sinus with arterial feeders from the internal carotid artery only in type B, meningeal branches of the external carotid artery in type C, and from both the internal

and external carotid arteries in type D. Thomas[16] and Wenderoth[17] have proposed variations on the original Barrow classification that are based on the pattern of venous drainage, which has implications for endovascular access and treatment. In rare circumstances, osteodural fistulae of the anterior or middle skull base can involve the cavernous sinus and present similarly.[18]

EVALUATION: CLINICAL PRESENTATION

Clinical presentation depends on CCF type, as well as the pattern of alteration of venous outflow from the cavernous sinus. By its nature, direct CCF typically present acutely with a combination of acute onset headache, retro-orbital pain, chemosis, proptosis, ocular bruit, and oculomotor dysfunction.[8,19–21] Diplopia due to oculomotor palsy is common.[8] Rarely, subarachnoid hemorrhage (SAH) may be seen. Although SAH is typically unrelated in the setting of trauma, if a giant cavernous segment aneurysm escapes the confines of the cavernous sinus dura, rupture may result in both CCF and SAH.[20,22,23]

The presentation of indirect CCF is often more insidious, and as a result, diagnosis is often delayed as the patient is worked up for more common diseases that present with similar ocular symptoms, such as infectious or inflammatory conjunctivitis or thyroid disease.[8] Indirect CCF with anterior drainage, or reversal of flow in the superior and/or inferior ophthalmic veins, typically present with arterialization of the conjunctival and episcleral veins delimited by the limbus, proptosis, decreased visual acuity from ischemic injury to the optic nerve as a result of increased intraorbital pressure, and oculomotor dysmotility from palsies of one or more cranial nerves 3, 4, and 6.[1,8,11,16,19–21] Facial pain from compression of the V1 and/or V2 divisions of the trigeminal nerve are rarer but reported.[24] Fistulae that drain retrograde into cortical veins may present with subarachnoid or intraparenchymal hemorrhage or alterations of cognition or personality as a consequence of intracranial venous hypertension.[25,26] Pulse-synchronous tinnitus is a common presenting symptom irrespective of venous drainage pattern.[8,16,27]

EVALUATION: IMAGING

Typical imaging workup for a suspected CCF, irrespective of subtype, requires vessel imaging. Computed tomography angiography (CTA) is a common first-line modality, but when the clinical suspicion is high for an indirect CCF, time-resolved magnetic resonance angiography has been demonstrated to provide excellent spatial and temporal

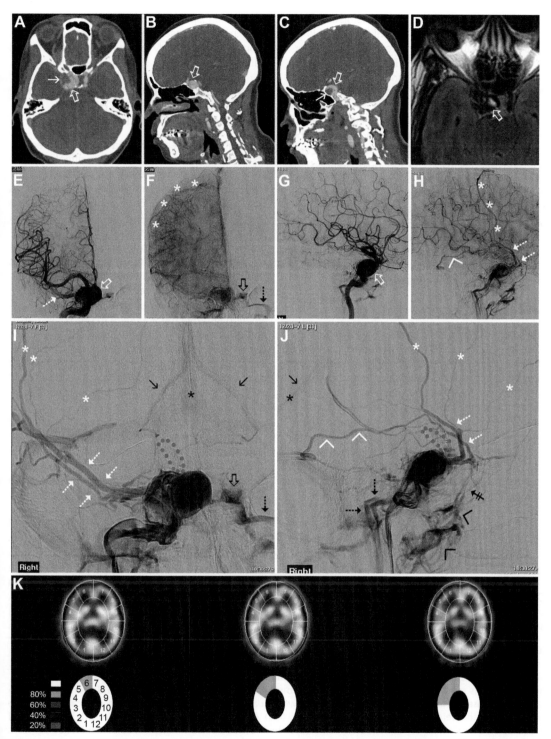

Fig. 1. Case example of a 47-year-old patient with a ruptured, giant, cavernous segment, ICA aneurysm with resultant direct CCF. (*A–D*) CTA and MRI demonstrated a partially thrombosed, giant, cavernous segment, right ICA aneurysm. Thrombus is demarcated by the solid white arrow, whereas the filling component is highlighted by the white, open arrow. (*E, F*) Anteroposterior (AP) view of the right ICA injection on DSA demonstrates a ruptured giant aneurysm of the cavernous segment of the ICA (*open arrow*), with carotid cavernous fistulation. Drainage is via the bilateral cavernous sinuses. The arterial phase (*E*) reveals shunting into the Sylvian veins (*white, dashed arrow*), whereas the capillary/early venous phase (*F*) shows reflux into a large, frontal cortical

resolution to characterize these fistulae.[28–30] A distinct aneurysm is sometimes distinguishable on axial imaging in the setting of direct CCF. Characteristics of CCF on axial imaging include dilation of the cavernous sinus, superior and/or inferior orbital veins (SOV and/or IOV), or cortical veins entering the cavernous or sphenoparietal sinuses.[27,31–33] Edema within the extraocular muscles and orbital fat stranding may be present and indicates intraorbital venous hypertension.[34] Digital subtraction cerebral angiography (DSA) is the gold standard to characterize CCFs, their arterial supply, venous drainage pattern, and alterations in orbital and intracranial hemodynamics and develop a treatment plan. When completing DSA in the evaluation of CCF, it is critical that the bilateral ECA, ICA, and VA are injected, as indirect CCF can be supplied by dural branches of any of the aforementioned arteries, even from the contralateral side.

APPROACH

The first consideration in treating CCFs is the subtype. In general, direct CCF are treated by reconstruction of the ICA when possible or necessary. Indirect CCF are overwhelmingly treated by endovascular techniques in the modern era. The goal of treatment of indirect CCF is complete obliteration of the point of shunting and the cavernous sinus. Spontaneous occlusion of indirect CCF is a rare but documented phenomenon.[20] In patients who are high risk for intervention, or in those who suffer from fistulae with extraordinarily slow flow, conservative management may be considered. Intermittent, daily, common carotid artery compression over a period of weeks to months has been demonstrated to promote complete thrombosis in select patients. In a small, highly selected cohort, 30% (7 of 23) of patients with indirect CCF and 17% (8 of 48) of patients with direct CCF went on to durable clinical and angiographic cure at 1 year.[35] When this technique is used, we suggest that patients use the contralateral hand

in case hemispheric ischemia becomes symptomatic, in which case the contralateral arm would drop and immediately restore flow to the affected hemisphere.

THERAPEUTIC OPTIONS: DIRECT CAROTID CAVERNOUS FISTULAE, TECHNIQUES, OUTCOMES, COMPLICATIONS

The first step in treatment of a direct CCF, regardless of cause, is to determine if the affected ICA is necessary to support adequate perfusion of the ipsilateral cerebral hemisphere. To do so, a balloon test occlusion (BTO) is completed, during which the ipsilateral ICA is temporarily occluded with a deflatable balloon, and the patient is clinically tested at predetermined intervals to assess for new neurologic symptoms referable to that hemisphere. Studies have demonstrated that the addition of various CT techniques that assess cerebral blood flow and perfusion during the balloon inflation improve the accuracy to predict ischemic complications if permanent sacrifice of that ICA is undertaken. Across series, the rate of ischemic complications, temporary or permanent, ranges from 0% to 22% in patients who pass a clinical and radionucleotide BTO who subsequently undergo carotid sacrifice.[36–38]

Our preference is to reconstruct the affected ICA whenever feasible to limit the risk of delayed ischemic complications or formation of intracranial aneurysms of the contralateral anterior circulation because of augmented hemodynamic stress due to increased demand. Reconstruction is generally achieved through a combination of luminal restoration through stenting with adjunctive coiling of the aneurysm, if the anatomy of the aneurysm is reasonably maintained, or combination of transarterial or transvenous cavernous sinus coiling, if the aneurysm is structurally compromised and will no longer hold coils. Stenting to reestablish the ICA lumen can be achieved with a flow-diverting stent.[39] The advantage of a flow-diverting stent is

vein (*white asterisks*), the contralateral cavernous sinus (*black, open arrow*), and the contralateral IPS (*black, dashed arrow*). (G, H) Arterial and late arterial phase lateral. Right ICA angiograms demonstrate the ruptured, giant cavernous segment aneurysm (*open, white arrow*) with preserved antegrade flow and shunting into the cavernous sinuses, with reflux into the Sylvian veins (*white, dashed arrows*), then into frontal cortical veins (*white asterisks*) and the vein of Labbé (*white arrowhead*). (I, J) AP (I) and lateral (J) angiograms after supraclinoid balloon inflation. Outline of the balloon is demarcated by the blue dotted outline. An arterial injection confirms complete, temporary ICA occlusion and isolates the venous drainage pattern of the direct CCF. Drainage is via the bilateral cavernous sinuses (*open black arrow*) with cortical venous reflux both to the Sylvian venous system (*white, dashed arrows*) and to cortical veins (*white asterisks*), including the vein of Labbé (*white arrowheads*), as well as the Galenic system (*black asterisk*) via the basal veins of Rosenthal (*black arrow*). Drainage through the dural sinus system is through the bilateral IPS (*dashed black arrows*) and the sphenoparietal sinuses (*hatched, black arrow*) to the pterygoid plexuses (*black arrowheads*). (K) Before clinical failure and balloon deflation, Technetium-99 was given intravenously, and single-photon emission computed tomography (SPECT) revealed a 10% diminution in right frontal lobe relative to the left (cortical segments 4–6).

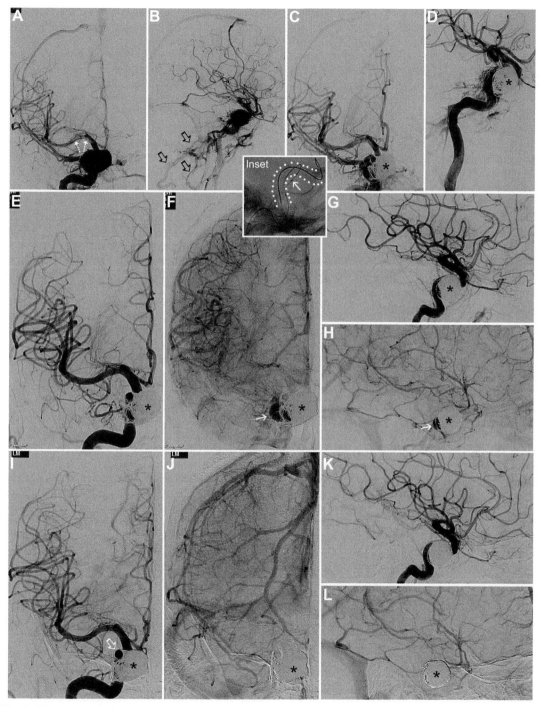

Fig. 2. Treatment of the ruptured, giant, cavernous segment ICA aneurysm with resultant direct CCF by flow diversion, with adjunctive transarterial flow diversion. (*A, B*) Treatment was conducted several days after the initial workup and balloon test occlusion described in **Fig. 1**. In the interim, increasing sump effect altered antegrade flow through the diseased segment with increased contribution from collaterals via the circle of Willis, as demonstrated by streaming, unopacified blood from the supraclinoid ICA to the MCA (*dashed, white arrows*) and accentuated drainage through occipital and paraspinous venous plexus collaterals via the IPS at the sigmoid-jugular bulb transition (*open black arrows*). The aneurysm was treated with two telescoping flow-diverting stents (inset—*white dotted outline*) with the coiling microcatheter jailed in the aneurysm (inset—*white arrow*). (*C, D*) Immediate posttreatment angiography revealed slowed but persistent flow through the fistula. The coil mass is

familiarity with the device among neuro-interventionists, deliverability, and on-label use. The disadvantage is the porosity of the stent, which requires adjunctive coiling in most instances to completely treat the direct CCF. Despite coiling, flow demand through the fistula may result in incomplete obliteration. Off-label use of covered stents,[40,41] such as those approved for coronary artery rupture, are increasingly used to treat direct CCF but suffer from stiffness that often limits the ability to deliver the device sufficiently across the ICA aneurysm or injury. The advantage of a covered stent is immediate and reliable closure of the fistulous point. High-flow bypass is reserved for patients who cannot undergo carotid sacrifice due to a failed BTO in whom endovascular reconstruction is not possible.

THERAPEUTIC OPTIONS: INDIRECT CAROTID CAVERNOUS FISTULAE, TECHNIQUES, OUTCOMES, COMPLICATIONS

Today, indirect CCF are near exclusively treated by endovascular techniques with the goal of complete disconnection of the fistula by obliterating the portion of the cavernous sinus into which the shunt enters. Historically, and in cases in which endovascular access has been exhausted, surgical exposure of the cavernous sinus with packing remains an effective treatment option.[42–44] Unlike many dAVFs, in which transarterial embolization is common and effective, transarterial embolization of cavernous sinus dAVF is fraught with danger due to the risk of nontargeted embolization to the retina or ICA through skull base collaterals from common arterial feeders to indirect CCF.[45] Examples include the recurrent meningeal branch of the middle meningeal artery to the lacrimal artery or the artery of foramen rotundum to the inferolateral trunk. Detachable coils are the traditional embolic material used to treat indirect CCF; however, liquid embolic agents such as ethylene vinyl alcohol are being increasingly used with an acceptable safety profile.[46] The advantage of liquid embolic agents over coils is their ability to pervade the complex trabeculae of the cavernous sinus and for the operator to make adequately dense the embolic cast in the area of the fistulous connection. Access to the cavernous sinus for treatment of indirect CCF is typically transvenous. The most direct and accessible route is via the inferior petrosal sinus (IPS), but in many instances, high-flow venopathy has led to occlusion of the ipsilateral IPS. An occluded IPS can be successfully bored through in about 50% of cases.[47,48] In other instances, the contralateral IPS, either superior petrosal sinus (SPS) or cavernous sinus access via the facial vein to the SOV can be achieved. Traversing the venous rete that often exists at the superior aspect of the orbit where the angular vein transitions to the SOV is often challenging. Catheterization of the SPS is easier from the contralateral jugular vein as the trajectory from the transverse sinus to the SPS ostium is straight from the contralateral approach and highly acute from the ipsilateral side. When the cavernous sinus is completely isolated, ultrasound-guided access to the SOV or direct cannulation via surgical exposure in combination with oculoplastic surgery colleagues is possible. However, the steep upward trajectory to access the SOV via a percutaneous approach given its position in the orbit, followed by the steep decline in trajectory into the cavernous sinus, makes this approach technically challenging.[49] Far simpler is transorbital, trans-superior orbital fissure, direct puncture of the cavernous sinus, a method routinely used in our institution with low morbidity with a high rate of complete occlusion and substantially reduced fluoroscopy time as compared with more traditional embolization strategies.[46,50,51]

Fistulae that are incompletely embolized, but through which flow has been substantially reduced, can be safely treated with intravenous epsilon-aminocaproic acid, which has been demonstrated to increase the rate of subsequent complete occlusion on follow-up angiography from 34% to 55% without increased risk of thromboembolic complications.[52]

Stereotactic radiosurgery (SRS) is limited to treatment of indirect CCF only and is typically reserved for patients who have either failed surgical or endovascular intervention or who are poor candidates to undergo anesthesia. Obliteration rates are typically lower than that for surgery or endovascular treatment; although, indirect CCF are more likely to undergo complete obliteration than other intracranial dAVFs following SRS.[53,54] In a systematic review of 729 patients, the cure

---

highlighted by the black asterisk. (E–H) Six-week follow-up angiography showed no early phase CCF shunting [(E) AP; (G) lateral), but capillary into venous phase angiography revealed persistent filling of the cavernous sinus with prolonged stagnation of contrast [white arrow, (F) AP; (H) lateral). (I–L) Three-month follow-up angiography revealed complete occlusion of the aneurysm and CCF in all phases of angiography [(I) arterial phase AP; (J) venous phase AP; (K) arterial phase lateral; (L) venous phase lateral) with complete luminal reconstruction (open, white arrow).

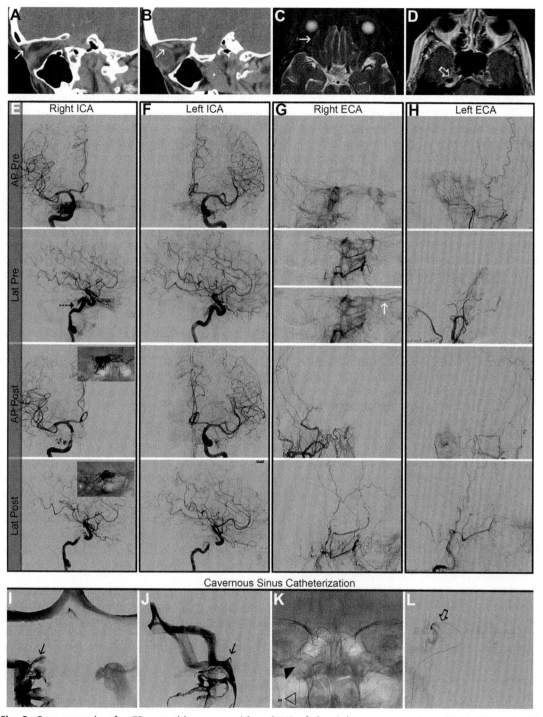

Fig. 3. Case example of a 73-year-old woman with a dAVF of the right cavernous sinus. (*A–D*) CTA and MRI demonstrated dilation of the right SOV (*white arrows*) and expansion and enhancement of the right cavernous sinus (*open, white arrow*). (*E–H*) On DSA, a right cavernous sinus dAVF was revealed with arterial supply from dural branches of the cavernous ICA bilaterally [(*E*) and (*F*) AP preoperative [Pre] and lateral Pre (Lat Pre)], multiple dural branches of the right ECA system, including the middle meningeal and accessory meningeal arteries as well as the artery of foramen rotundum [(*G*) AP Pre and Lat Pre], and the contralateral ascending pharyngeal artery [(*H*) AP Pre and Lat Pre]. Venous drainage was via the cavernous sinuses bilaterally without outflow into the left IPS and right SPS with reversal of flow in the right SOV (*white arrow*) and cortical veins that ultimately drain to the Galenic system via the basal veins of Rosenthal bilaterally [(*E*)–(*H*) AP Pre and Lat Pre]. Notably, the

rate for SRS for patients with indirect CCF was 73% versus 58% for all others.[53] The complication rate of SRS is low.[53,54]

The cure rate for endovascular treatment of CCF, whether direct or indirect, is high, with most modern series approaching 90%.[49,52,55–58] Complications of treatment tend to be thrombo-embolic, either to the brain or retina. Transient or permanent worsening of cranial neuropathies is commonly reported, as is further deterioration of vision, either due to ischemia of the optic nerve due to compression or due to pervasive intraorbital hypertension.[7,8,20,46–48,51,53–60] Transient worsening of symptoms is reported to be as high as nearly 50%.[60] Intracranial hemorrhage from non-targeted embolization into affected cortical veins with resultant venous hypertension, stroke, and hemorrhagic conversion is also reported.[61] Provocation of the trigeminal cardiac reflex is possible during infusion of the microcatheter with dimethyl sulfoxide (DMSO) when using ethylene vinyl alcohol.[48] To avoid bradycardia, which can progress to asystole, slow infusion of the DMSO is essential, as is a team approach with anesthesia colleagues to assure their preparedness with counteracting medications, such as atropine. Transorbital puncture may result in retrobulbar hematoma, which if not recognized and immediately treated with a canthotomy, may exacerbate intraorbital hypertension and vision loss.[46,49,51,59] SRS may be complicated by optic neuritis or intracranial radiation necrosis from radiation toxicity.[29]

CASE STUDY/PRESENTATION: DIRECT CAROTID CAVERNOUS FISTULAE

The patient was a 47-year-old woman with limited medical history who presented with acute onset right frontal headache and retro-orbital pain, ophthalmoplegia, proptosis, and a mydriatic, nonreactive right pupil. The patient wore glasses for refraction correction at baseline, and visual acuity was 20/30 in the left eye and 20/200 in the right on presentation. Sensation was decreased in the V1 distribution. Otherwise, the neurologic and systemic examination were normal.

Noncontrast-enhanced CT demonstrated hyperdensity in the right cavernous sinus with no other abnormalities. CTA and MRI demonstrated

a partially thrombosed, giant, cavernous segment, right ICA aneurysm, which was later confirmed on DSA. DSA demonstrated the aneurysm with preserved antegrade flow into the brain, early filling of the cavernous sinuses bilaterally, and venous drainage through the right SOV, SPS, multiple cortical veins, and the bilateral IPS and pterygoid plexuses. The patient failed a subsequent BTO, during which, after 15 minutes of balloon inflation, she developed left facial and upper extremity sensory changes and a pronator drift. The balloon was immediately deflated with reversal of symptoms. Technetium-99 had already been given and single-photon emission computed tomography (SPECT) revealed a 10% diminution in the right frontal lobe. Baseline SPECT the following day confirmed symmetric perfusion, indicating that sacrifice of the right ICA would not be clinically tolerated (**Fig. 1**). Therefore, a reconstructive approach was taken. A completely transarterial approach was taken. Telescoping flow-diverting stents were placed, and a coiling catheter was jailed in the cavernous sinus. Coiling was completed until the coiling catheter was kicked out of the cavernous sinus. Shunting was slowed but persistent immediately after treatment.

Follow-up DSA at 6 weeks demonstrated additional slowing of the direct CCF. DSA at 3 months showed complete resolution of the CCF with reconstruction of the cavernous segment of the right ICA (**Fig. 2**).

As of 4 months after treatment, her cranial nerve 3, 4, 5, and 6 palsies had substantially improved. Proptosis had resolved. Visual acuity in the left eye was 20/20 and 20/30 in the right. Intraocular pressure was normal. Mild diplopia was noted on certain gaze and was manageable with lid taping. The patient refused referral for strabismus surgery as her diplopia did not negatively affect her daily life.

CASE STUDY/PRESENTATION: INDIRECT CAROTID CAVERNOUS FISTULAE WITH OCCLUDED INFERIOR PETROSAL SINUS

The patient was a 73-year-old woman with a past medical history significant only for hypertension who presented to clinic with a 2-month history of lancinating, right retro-orbital pain and diplopia. She had been treated with oral anticoagulation

ipsilateral IPS was occluded as it exits the cavernous sinus [(*E*) Lat Pre; (*I*) and (*J*) black, dashed arrow]. The fistula was treated with transvenous embolization with ethylene vinyl alcohol copolymer via navigation of the unopacified right IPS [(*K*), (*L*)—open arrow: tip of long sheath in the proximal jugular vein; black arrowhead: tip of guide catheter in the stump of the IPS; black, open arrow: tip of the microcatheter at the point of the fistula in the posterior aspect of the right cavernous sinus with microinjection for confirmation of catheter placement). Complete occlusion was achieved [(*E*)–(*H*) AP postoperative [Post] and Lat Post; insets demonstrate the final embolic cast).

before her presentation for a presumed cavernous sinus thrombosis. Her examination was normal, except the following abnormalities: 20/25 visual acuity on the right as compared with 20/20 on the left and a right abducens palsy. The remainder of her detailed neuro-ophthalmologic examination was normal. Her previous CTA of the orbits and MRI demonstrated subtle findings most consistent with an indirect CCF, and therefore, her anticoagulation was stopped. These axial imaging modalities showed an asymmetrically dilated right SOV and early enhancement of the right cavernous sinus. This constellation of clinical and radiographic findings led to DSA, which confirmed the indirect CCF.

On DSA, a right cavernous sinus dAVF was revealed with arterial supply from dural branches of the cavernous ICA bilaterally, multiple dural branches of the right ECA system, including the middle meningeal and accessory meningeal arteries as well as the artery of foramen rotundum, and the meningeal trunk of the contralateral ascending pharyngeal artery (Barrow type D). Venous drainage was via the cavernous sinuses bilaterally without outflow into the left IPS and right SPS with reversal of flow in the right SOV and cortical veins, which ultimately drain to the Galenic system via the basal veins of Rosenthal bilaterally. Notably, the ipsilateral IPS was occluded. The fistula was treated with transvenous embolization with ethylene vinyl alcohol copolymer via navigation of the unopacified right IPS. Complete occlusion was achieved (**Fig. 3**).

At follow-up, the retroorbital pain had resolved completely. The abducens palsy did not improve, and a new partial third nerve palsy, characterized by moderate ptosis, was noted. Her diplopia was being effectively managed with eye patching.

SUMMARY

CCF are arteriovenous shunts that abnormally arterialize the cavernous sinus. CCF are divided into direct, or a connection from the ICA into the cavernous sinus, most typically from a ruptured aneurysm or trauma, and indirect, which are essentially dural fistulae of the cavernous sinus wall. Treatment is directed toward the specific subtype and is overwhelmingly endovascular in the modern era. Most CCF can be safely and effectively managed through endovascular therapy.

CLINICS CARE POINTS

- Treatment of CCF is determined by the subtype of fistula.

- Direct CCF are treated by either deconstructive or reconstructive techniques depending on whether the affected ICA is required to sufficiently perfuse the ipsilateral cerebral hemisphere.

- If the patient passes a BOT, ICA sacrifice is often the most straightforward treatment of a direct CCF. If the BTO is failed, a reconstructive approach, typically with flow diversion and coiling, is required.

- Indirect CCF, which represent dural fistulae of the cavernous sinus wall, are most often treated with transvenous embolization in the modern era.

- SRS is reserved for cases of indirect CCF that are not completed obliterated by embolization. The cure rate for SRS of indirect CCF is higher than that of dAVF in other locations.

DISCLOSURE

The authors have no conflict of interest to disclose. No extramural funding was used in the production of this submission.

REFERENCES

1. Barrow DL, Spector RH, Braun IF, et al. Classification and treatment of spontaneous carotid-cavernous sinus fistulas. J Neurosurg 1985;62(2):248–56.
2. Travers B. A case of Aneurism by Anastomosis in the Orbit, cured by the Ligature of the common Carotid Artery. Med Chir Trans 1811;2:1–420.
3. Aubry M. Tumeur erectile de l'Orbite; pulsations; bruit de souffle; erreur de diagnostic; dilatation de la veine ophthalmique. Gazette des Hôpitaux; 1864.
4. Rivington W. A Case of Pulsating Tumour of the Left Orbit, consequent upon a Fracture of the Base of the Skull, Cured by Ligature of the Left Common Carotid Artery, subsequently to Injection of Perchloride of Iron, after Digital Compression and other means of Treatment had failed; with Remarks, and an Appendix containing a Chronological Resume of Recorded Cases of Intra-orbital Aneurism. Med Chir Trans 1875;58:183–298.
5. Rhoton AL Jr. The cavernous sinus, the cavernous venous plexus, and the carotid collar. Neurosurgery 2002;51(4 Suppl):S375–410.
6. Biffl WL, Moore EE, Offner PJ, et al. Blunt carotid arterial injuries: implications of a new grading scale. J Trauma 1999;47(5):845–53.
7. Fabian TS, Woody JD, Ciraulo DL, et al. Posttraumatic carotid cavernous fistula: frequency analysis of signs, symptoms, and disability outcomes after angiographic embolization. J Trauma 1999;47(2):275–81.

8. Williams ZR. Carotid-Cavernous Fistulae: A Review of Clinical Presentation, Therapeutic Options, and Visual Prognosis. Int Ophthalmol Clin 2018;58(2): 271–94.

9. Li C, Zhu H, Zong X, et al. Experience of trans-nasal endoscopic surgery for pituitary tumors in a single center in China: Surgical results in a cohort of 2032 patients, operated between 2006 and 2018. Clin Neurol Neurosurg 2020;197:106176.

10. Porras JL, Rowan NR, Mukherjee D. Endoscopic Endonasal Skull Base Surgery Complication Avoidance: A Contemporary Review. Brain Sci 2022; 12(12). https://doi.org/10.3390/brainsci12121685.

11. Guest W, Krings T. Transvenous Approaches to Embolization of Dural Arteriovenous Fistulae of the Cavernous Sinus. J Neuroendovasc Ther 2022; 16(2):63–73.

12. Lawton MT, Jacobowitz R, Spetzler RF. Redefined role of angiogenesis in the pathogenesis of dural arteriovenous malformations. J Neurosurg 1997; 87(2):267–74.

13. Terada T, Tsuura M, Komai N, et al. The role of angiogenic factor bFGF in the development of dural AVFs. Acta Neurochir 1996;138(7):877–83.

14. LaHue SC, Kim H, Pawlikowska L, et al. Frequency and characteristics associated with inherited thrombophilia in patients with intracranial dural arteriovenous fistula. J Neurosurg 2018;130(4):1346–50.

15. Terada T, Higashida RT, Halbach VV, et al. Development of acquired arteriovenous fistulas in rats due to venous hypertension. J Neurosurg 1994;80(5): 884–9.

16. Thomas AJ, Chua M, Fusco M, et al. Proposal of Venous Drainage-Based Classification System for Carotid Cavernous Fistulae With Validity Assessment in a Multicenter Cohort. Neurosurgery 2015; 77(3):380–5 [discussion: 385].

17. Wenderoth J. Proposal for an improved classification system for cavernous sinus dural arteriovenous fistula (CS-DAVF). J Neurointerv Surg 2017;9(3):220–4.

18. Howard BM, Manupipatpong S, Dion JE, et al. Classification and Management Considerations for Intraosseous Dural Arteriovenous Fistulae. Neurosurgery 2023;93(2):387–98.

19. Debrun GM, Davis KR, Nauta HJ, et al. Treatment of carotid cavernous fistulae or cavernous aneurysms associated with a persistent trigeminal artery: report of three cases. AJNR Am J Neuroradiol 1988;9(4): 749–55.

20. Ellis JA, Goldstein H, Connolly ES Jr, et al. Carotid-cavernous fistulas. Neurosurg Focus 2012;32(5):E9.

21. Gupta AK, Purkayastha S, Krishnamoorthy T, et al. Endovascular treatment of direct carotid cavernous fistulae: a pictorial review. Neuroradiology 2006; 48(11):831–9.

22. Wiebers DO, Whisnant JP, Huston J 3rd, et al. Unruptured intracranial aneurysms: natural history, clinical outcome, and risks of surgical and endovascular treatment. Lancet 2003;362(9378):103–10.

23. Liang W, Xiaofeng Y, Weiguo L, et al. Traumatic carotid cavernous fistula accompanying basilar skull fracture: a study on the incidence of traumatic carotid cavernous fistula in the patients with basilar skull fracture and the prognostic analysis about traumatic carotid cavernous fistula. J Trauma 2007; 63(5):1014–20 [discussion: 1020].

24. Fukutome K, Nakagawa I, Park HS, et al. Resolution of Trigeminal Neuralgia After Transvenous Embolization of a Cavernous Sinus Dural Arteriovenous Fistula. World Neurosurg 2017;98:880 e5–e880 e8.

25. Borden JA, Wu JK, Shucart WA. A proposed classification for spinal and cranial dural arteriovenous fistulous malformations and implications for treatment. J Neurosurg 1995;82(2):166–79.

26. Cognard C, Gobin YP, Pierot L, et al. Cerebral dural arteriovenous fistulas: clinical and angiographic correlation with a revised classification of venous drainage. Radiology 1995;194(3):671–80.

27. Robertson A, Nicolaides AR, Taylor RH. Spontaneous carotico-cavernous fistula presenting as pulsatile tinnitus. J Laryngol Otol 1999;113(8):744–6.

28. Sakamoto S, Shibukawa M, Kiura Y, et al. Evaluation of dural arteriovenous fistulas of cavernous sinus before and after endovascular treatment using time-resolved MR angiography. Neurosurg Rev 2010;33(2):217–22 [discussion: 222–3].

29. Wu CA, Yang HC, Hu YS, et al. Venous outflow restriction as a predictor of cavernous sinus dural arteriovenous fistula obliteration after Gamma Knife surgery. J Neurosurg 2019;1–8. https://doi.org/10. 3171/2018.9.JNS182040.

30. Grossberg JA, Howard BM, Saindane AM. The use of contrast-enhanced, time-resolved magnetic resonance angiography in cerebrovascular pathology. Neurosurg Focus 2019;47(6):E3.

31. Hu YS, Guo WY, Lin CJ, et al. Magnetic resonance imaging as a single diagnostic tool for verifying radiosurgery outcomes of cavernous sinus dural arteriovenous fistula. Eur J Radiol 2020;125: 108866.

32. Jindal G, Miller T, Raghavan P, et al. Imaging Evaluation and Treatment of Vascular Lesions at the Skull Base. Radiol Clin North Am 2017;55(1):151–66.

33. Rahman WT, Griauzde J, Chaudhary N, et al. Neurovascular emergencies: imaging diagnosis and neurointerventional treatment. Emerg Radiol 2017; 24(2):183–93.

34. Biousse V, Mendicino ME, Simon DJ, et al. The ophthalmology of intracranial vascular abnormalities. Am J Ophthalmol 1998;125(4):527–44.

35. Higashida RT, Hieshima GB, Halbach VV, et al. Closure of carotid cavernous sinus fistulae by external compression of the carotid artery and jugular vein. Acta Radiol Suppl 1986;369:580–3.

36. Segal DH, Sen C, Bederson JB, et al. Predictive value of balloon test occlusion of the internal carotid artery. Skull Base Surg 1995;5(2):97–107.

37. Sivakumaran R, Mohamed AZ, Akhunbay-Fudge CY, et al. Internal Carotid Artery Test Balloon Occlusion Using Single Photon Emission Computed Tomography Scan in the Management of Complex Cerebral Aneurysms and Skull Base Tumors: A 20-Year Review. World Neurosurg 2020;139:e32–7.

38. Yamamoto Y, Nishiyama Y, Toyama Y, et al. Preliminary results of Tc-99m ECD SPECT to evaluate cerebral collateral circulation during balloon test occlusion. Clin Nucl Med 2002;27(9):633–7.

39. Stamatopoulos T, Anagnostou E, Plakas S, et al. Treatment of carotid cavernous sinus fistulas with flow diverters. A case report and systematic review. Interv Neuroradiol 2022;28(1):70–83.

40. Madan A, Mujic A, Daniels K, et al. Traumatic carotid artery-cavernous sinus fistula treated with a covered stent. Report of two cases. J Neurosurg 2006; 104(6):969–73.

41. Morsi RZ, Thind S, Chahine A, et al. The use of PK Papyrus covered coronary stent for carotid reconstruction: an initial institutional experience. J Neurointerv Surg 2024. https://doi.org/10.1136/jnis-2023-021226.

42. Isamat F, Ferrer E, Twose J. Direct intracavernous obliteration of high-flow carotid-cavernous fistulas. J Neurosurg 1986;65(6):770–5.

43. Kosarchuk J, Patel S, Dent W, et al. Open Surgical Obliteration of Three Indirect Carotid-Cavernous Fistulas. Oper Neurosurg (Hagerstown) 2024. https://doi.org/10.1227/ons.0000000000001038.

44. Parkinson D. Direct obliteration of carotid-cavernous fistulas. J Neurosurg 1987;66(6):948.

45. Geibprasert S, Pongpech S, Armstrong D, et al. Dangerous extracranial-intracranial anastomoses and supply to the cranial nerves: vessels the neuro-interventionalist needs to know. AJNR Am J Neuroradiol 2009;30(8):1459–68.

46. Wenderoth J. Novel approaches to access and treatment of cavernous sinus dural arteriovenous fistula (CS-DAVF): case series and review of the literature. J Neurointerv Surg 2017;9(3):290–6.

47. Meyers PM, Halbach VV, Dowd CF, et al. Dural carotid cavernous fistula: definitive endovascular management and long-term follow-up. Am J Ophthalmol 2002;134(1):85–92.

48. Wang Y, Du B, Zhang J, et al. Embolization of cavernous sinus dural arteriovenous fistula via inferior petrosal sinus: anatomical basis and management practicability. Int J Clin Exp Med 2014;7(9): 3045–52.

49. Phan K, Xu J, Leung V, et al. Orbital Approaches for Treatment of Carotid Cavernous Fistulas: A Systematic Review. World Neurosurg 2016;96:243–51.

50. Narayanan S, Murchison AP, Wojno TH, et al. Percutaneous trans-superior orbital fissure embolization of carotid-cavernous fistulas: technique and preliminary results. Ophthalmic Plast Reconstr Surg 2009; 25(4):309–13.

51. Teng MM, Lirng JF, Chang T, et al. Embolization of carotid cavernous fistula by means of direct puncture through the superior orbital fissure. Radiology 1995;194(3):705–11.

52. Howard BM, Grossberg JA, Prater A, et al. Incompletely obliterated cranial arteriovenous fistulae are safely and effectively treated with adjuvant epsilon-aminocaproic acid. J Neurointerv Surg 2018;10(7): 698–703.

53. Chen CJ, Lee CC, Ding D, et al. Stereotactic radiosurgery for intracranial dural arteriovenous fistulas: a systematic review. J Neurosurg 2015;122(2): 353–62.

54. Hung YC, Mohammed N, Kearns KN, et al. Stereotactic Radiosurgery for Cavernous Sinus Versus Noncavernous Sinus Dural Arteriovenous Fistulas: Outcomes and Outcome Predictors. Neurosurgery 2020;86(5):676–84.

55. Gemmete JJ, Chaudhary N, Pandey A, et al. Treatment of carotid cavernous fistulas. Curr Treat Options Neurol 2010;12(1):43–53.

56. Chen CJ, Buell TJ, Ding D, et al. Intervention for unruptured high-grade intracranial dural arteriovenous fistulas: a multicenter study. J Neurosurg 2022; 136(4):962–70.

57. Ng PP, Higashida RT, Cullen S, et al. Endovascular strategies for carotid cavernous and intracerebral dural arteriovenous fistulas. Neurosurg Focus 2003;15(4):ECP1.

58. Yoshida K, Melake M, Oishi H, et al. Transvenous embolization of dural carotid cavernous fistulas: a series of 44 consecutive patients. AJNR Am J Neuroradiol 2010;31(4):651–5.

59. Elhammady MS, Peterson EC, Aziz-Sultan MA. Onyx embolization of a carotid cavernous fistula via direct transorbital puncture. J Neurosurg 2011;114(1): 129–32.

60. Roy D, Raymond J. The role of transvenous embolization in the treatment of intracranial dural arteriovenous fistulas. Neurosurgery 1997;40(6):1133–41 [discussion: 1141–4].

61. Lee RJ, Chen CF, Hsu SW, et al. Cerebellar hemorrhage and subsequent venous infarction followed by incomplete transvenous embolization of dural carotid cavernous fistulas: a rare complication: case report. J Neurosurg 2008;108(6):1245–8.

Dural Arteriovenous Fistula

Kareem El Naamani, MD[a], Stavropoula I. Tjoumakaris, MD[a], Michael Reid Gooch, MD[a], Pascal Jabbour, MD[a],*

KEYWORDS

- Dural arteriovenous fistula • Diagnosis • Borden classification • Cognard classification • Surgery
- Embolization

KEY POINTS

- Dural arteriovenous fistulas are rare cerebrovascular entities that can cause significant morbidity and mortality if left untreated.
- Classification is essential for diagnosis and dictation of treatment options.
- The main goal of treatment is to disconnect the fistulous point.
- Treatment options vary according to the lesions' characteristics and the patients' comorbidities and range from conservative observation to open surgery.

INTRODUCTION

Dural arteriovenous fistulas (DAVFs) are abnormal connections between meningeal arteries and dural venous sinuses or subarachnoid veins.[1] These lesions can occur at any age, but usually present between 50 and 60 years of age.[2] When DAVFs are presented in adulthood, these lesions are considered acquired, while presentation in children is considered congenital.[2] DAVFs arise within the dura matter and the fistulous connection is located within the dural leaflet.[3] As such, these lesions can be spinal or intracranial. Intracranial DAVFs (CDAVFs) account for 10% to 15% of all intracranial arteriovenous malformations. The most common locations include the cavernous sinus, cribriform plate, transverse sigmoid sinus, and the tentorium. CDAVFs are supplied by any dural branch of the internal carotid artery or external carotid artery and drain into the dural veins/sinus or cortical/perimedullary veins.[4] Presenting symptoms of CDAVFs are highly variable and depend on the location and anatomy of the lesion. The most common presentation of CDAVFs is pulsatile tinnitus which is present in 60% of patients on presentation.[5,6] More aggressive lesions can present with intracranial hemorrhages and nonhemorrhagic neurologic defect such as progressive dementia, pseudotumor cerebri, parkinsonism, and cervical myelopathy due to intracranial venous hypertension.[6–9] Spinal DAVFs (SDAVFs) are the most frequent spinal vascular malformations accounting for 70% of spinal vascular lesions.[10] These lesions are located in within the neural foramen along the nerve root sleeve and are supplied from the dural branch of the radicular artery.[11] Most SDAVFs (>80%) are located between T6 and L2, 4% are located in the sacral spine, and 2% are high cervical lesions (at the level of the foramen magnum).[12,13] The most common presenting symptom of SDAVFs is progressive myelopathy due to venous congestion which leads to reduced intramedullary blood flow, ischemia, and cord dysfunction.[14] In this article, we will discuss classification systems, diagnostic modalities, and different treatment techniques for DAVFs.

[a] Department of Neurological Surgery, Thomas Jefferson University Hospital, Philadelphia, PA, USA

* Corresponding author. Division of Neurovascular Surgery and Endovascular Neurosurgery, Thomas Jefferson University Hospital, 901 Walnut Street, 3rd Floor, Philadelphia, PA 19107.

E-mail address: pascal.jabbour@jefferson.edu

Neurosurg Clin N Am 35 (2024) 331–342
https://doi.org/10.1016/j.nec.2024.02.005

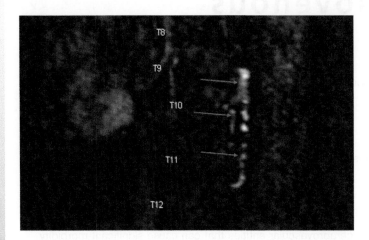

Fig. 1. Time-resolved imaging of contrast kinetics (TRICKS) MRI showing a spinal dural arteriovenous fistula (SDAVF) extending from spinal levels T9 to T11.

CLASSIFICATION SYSTEMS

When discussing DAVFs it is essential to use classification systems as these systems provide key information about drainage and size that dictates prognosis and treatment options.

In 1995, Borden and colleagues[15] proposed the Borden classification system for DAVFs which is based on drainage location solely and divided into 3 categories.

Borden Classification

Borden type I DAVFs: These DAVFs arise from an abnormal connection between a meningeal artery and a dural venous sinus or meningeal vein.[15] Because of the drainage to the dural venous sinus or meningeal vein from the brain or spine, the flow in these lesions is anterograde in nature. Thus, these lesions are considered benign with most patients presenting with tinnitus and only extremely rare cases result in hemorrhage or progress to higher grade DAVFs.[16,17]

Borden type II DAVFs: These DAVFs arise from an abnormal connection between a meningeal artery and the dural venous sinus intracranially or between a meningeal artery and the epidural venous plexus in the spine. However, due to high pressure that builds up in the sinus or epidural venous plexus, blood flows retrograde into the subarachnoid cortical veins intracranially or spinal perimedullary veins.[15] Because of the congestion of the subarachnoid veins, Borden type II DAVFs are considered aggressive and can cause hemorrhagic events and non-hemorrhagic neurologic defects. The annual rate of hemorrhage and neurologic defects ranges from 8.1% to 19.2% and 6.9% to 10.9%, respectively.[18–20]

Borden type III DAVFs: Unlike in previous grades, Borden type III DAVFs arise from an abnormal connection between a meningeal artery and a cortical vein intracranially or spinal perimedullary veins.[15] Similar to Borden type II DAVFs, these lesions also are aggressive and can cause hemorrhagic events and neurologic defects due to the retrograde venous flow.

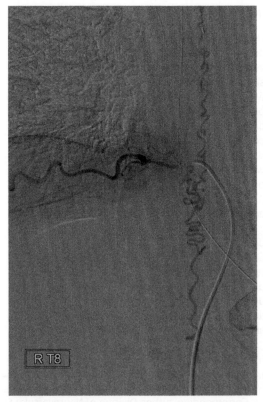

Fig. 2. Spinal digital subtraction angiography (anterior-posterior view) showing a spinal dural arteriovenous fistula (SDAVF) fed by spinal arteries at the level of T8.

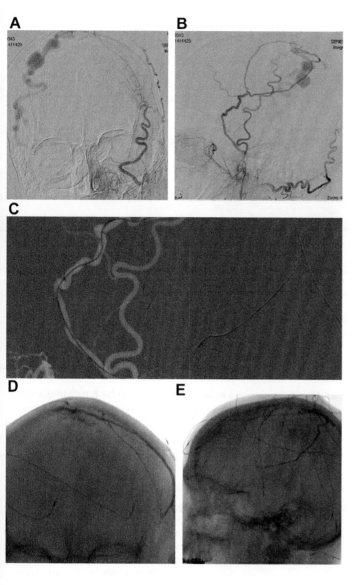

Fig. 3. (*A*) Angiography (anterior-posterior view) showing a cranial dural arteriovenous fistula (DAVF) fed by the left middle meningeal artery feeders with cortical venous drainage. (*B*) Angiography (lateral view) showing a cranial dural arteriovenous fistula (DAVF) fed by the left middle meningeal artery feeders with cortical venous drainage. (*C*) A scepter dual-lumen balloon microcatheter being navigated in the middle meningeal artery feeder. (*D*) Anterior-posterior X-ray view showing the Onyx cast. (*E*) Lateral X-ray view showing the Onyx cast.

Cognard Classification

Later in that same year, Cognard and colleagues[2] proposed a more detailed classification system that takes into consideration both the drainage location and size of the draining vein. (I, II, III, and IV).

Cognard type I DAVFs: Similar to Borden type I DAVFs, these lesions are benign and arise from an abnormal connection between a meningeal artery and a dural venous sinus or meningeal vein.[2] The flow in these lesions is a normal anterograde flow.

Cognard type II DAVFs: Similar to Borden type II DAVFs, these lesions arise from an abnormal connection between a meningeal artery and the

dural sinus where reflux takes place. Unlike the Borden classification, Cognard type II DAVFs are further divided into IIa, IIb, and IIa + IIb depending on the reflux destination.[2]

- In **type IIa DAVFs**, reflux flows only into the sinus.
- In **type IIb DAVFs**, reflux flows only into the cortical veins.
- In **type IIa + IIb DAVFs**, reflux flows into the sinus and cortical veins.

Cognard type III DAVFs: Similar to Borden type III DAVFs, these lesions arise from an abnormal connection between the meningeal artery and the cortical vein directly.[2] However,

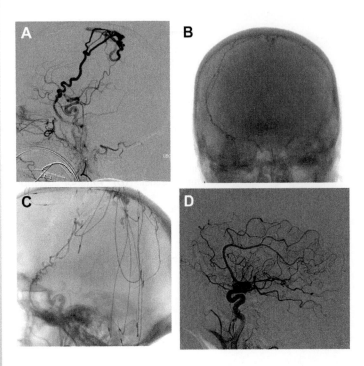

Fig. 4. (*A*) Angiography (lateral view) showing a cranial dural arteriovenous fistula (DAVF) fed by the left middle meningeal artery with cortical venous drainage. (*B*) Anterior-posterior X-ray view showing the Onyx cast. (*C*) Lateral X-ray view showing the Onyx cast. (*D*) Left common carotid artery angiography (lateral view) showing complete occlusion of the DAVF.

retrograde flow does not cause venous ectasia which is focal dilation of the vein due to arterialization.[2]

Cognard type IV DAVFs: These lesions are exactly similar to Cognard type III DAVFs; however, the only difference is the presence of venous ectasia which should be 5 mm in diameter and 3 times larger than the diameter of the draining vein.

Cognard type V DAVFs: These lesions are CDAVFs with exclusive drainage into the spinal perimedullary veins.[2]

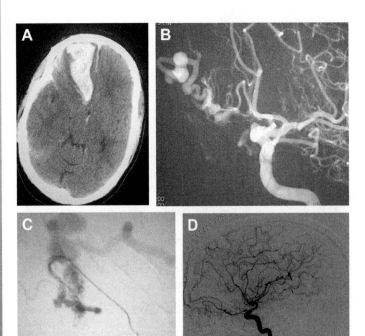

Fig. 5. (*A*) Axial brain computed tomography scan showing a right frontal hemorrhage. (*B*) Angiography (lateral view) showing an ethmoidal dural arteriovenous fistula (DAVF). (*C*) Superselective run in the ophthalmic artery distal to the take-off of the central retinal artery (*D*) Postoperative angiography (lateral view) showing complete occlusion of the DAVF.

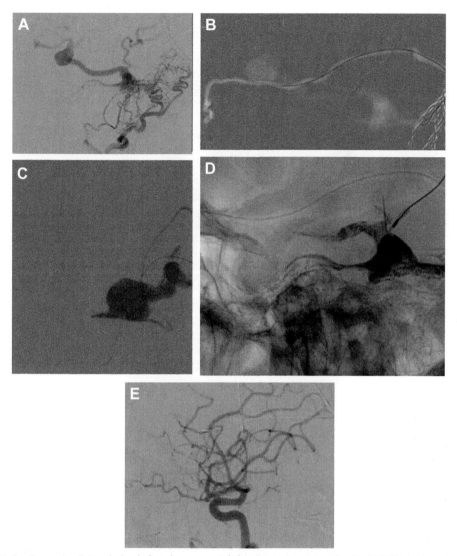

Fig. 6. (*A*) Angiography (lateral view) showing a cranial dural arteriovenous fistula (DAVF) fed by the occipital artery and middle meningeal artery with venous varices. (*B*) Navigation of the microcatheter through the middle meningeal artery. (*C*) Injection of Onyx. (*D*) X-ray showing the Onyx cast. (*E*) Postoperative angiography (lateral view) showing complete occlusion of the dural arteriovenous fistula (DAVF).

DIAGNOSIS

When diagnosing a DAVF, it is important to accurately localize the lesion, identify the number of feeding arteries and draining veins, and highlight the presence of cortical venous drainage and ectasia.[21] This information is essential for classification and deciding on a treatment modality.

Computed Tomography

Computed tomography (CT) scan is rarely used to diagnose DAVFs but rather is usually the initial radiographic evaluation in patients presenting with symptoms of hemorrhage.[22] CT scans can be used to detect DAVFs-related intracranial hemorrhages and vasogenic edema caused by venous hypertension.[22] Furthermore, this imaging modality does not provide accurate localization of the fistula as venous varices are usually the source of hemorrhage and are distant from the actual location of the lesion.[23]

MRI

Because of its superior resolution and ability to detect neighboring neurologic structures, an MRI can help in delineating a DAVF's anatomy.[22] Using

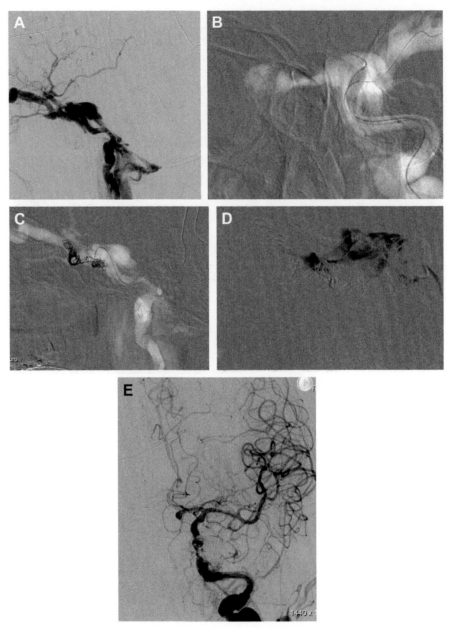

Fig. 7. (*A*) Angiography (lateral view) showing a cranial Barrow type A carotid cavernous fistula (CCF). (*B*) Balloon-assisted transarterial embolization. (*C*) Coiling of the CCF. (*D*) Adjunct Onyx embolization to coiling. (*E*) Postoperative angiography (anterior-posterior view) showing complete occlusion of the CCF.

T2-weighted imaging, arterialized draining veins and varices can be detected. Hyperintensities on T2-weighted imaging can suggest vasogenic edema.[24] T1-weighted imaging can further show venous ectasia, leptomeningeal and medullary vessel dilation, venous sinus occlusion/stenosis, and parenchymal enhancement.[25] Decreased apparent diffusion coefficient and a dynamic susceptibility contrast MRI can be used to identify retrograde cortical drainage.[26,27] Lastly, an MRI can be used to diagnose hydrocephalus and intracranial hemorrhage.

A new promising magnetic resonance sequence mainly used as a first-line noninvasive imaging screening for patients with suspected SDAVFs is the time-resolved imaging of contrast kinetics (TRICKS). The main idea behind the introduction of the TRICKS MRI is its ability to accurately detect the level of the SDAVF $\pm$ 1 level which can be used to guide a more specific spinal digital subtraction

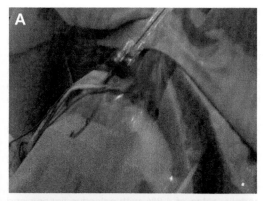

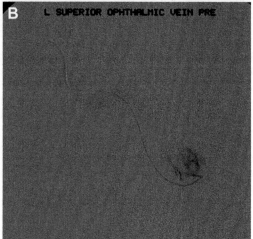

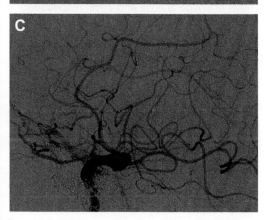

Fig. 8. (*A*) Superior ophthalmic vein approach for carotid cavernous fistula (CCF) treatment. (*B*) Microcatheter navigation from the superior orbital vein to the cavernous sinus. (*C*) Postoperative angiography (lateral view) showing complete occlusion of the CCF.

angiography (DSA) rather than catheterize all the spinal levels (**Fig. 1**).[28]

Digital Subtraction Angiography

A DSA remains the gold standard imaging modality for the diagnosis of DAVFs. Intracranially, a 6-

vessel DSA is necessary as some lesion may have bilateral supply (**Fig. 2**).[29] In SDAVFs, DSA-based diagnosis requires the catheterization of all intercostal arteries.[30] During the venous phase, it is important to assess venous anatomy, the presence of cortical venous drainage, and venous outflow (stenosis or occlusion).[21,29] The presence of tortuous and engorged veins during the venous phase is referred to as pseudophlebitic pattern which is seen in 81% of cortical venous drainage cases.[29] DSA also gives the option of superselective catheterization to accurately identify the point of convergence of the feeding artery and the origin of the draining vein.[22]

TREATMENT
Cranial Dural Arteriovenous Fistulas

Treatment options for DAVFs range from observation to endovascular treatment, surgical intervention, radiosurgery, and a combination of modalities based on several factors, some of which are patient-related (symptoms and demographics) and others are DAVF-related (dimensions, classification, and location). The primary objective of DAVF treatment is to obliterate the proximal segment of the draining vein.[31]

Conservative management
Borden type I and Cognard types I and IIa DAVFs without cortical venous drainage are considered benign lesions with an annual risk of new neurologic symptoms and mortality of 0% to 0.6% and 0%, respectively.[17,31–33] Because of this benign nature, these DAVFs are treated conservatively; however, prompt radiological assessment is warranted when patients develop new symptoms. Palliative treatment is usually offered to patients with disabling tinnitus, ophthalmologic symptoms, or headaches with the goal of improving quality of life. The goal of palliative treatment is to reduce the degree of shunting to address the disabling symptoms in cases where the treatment-related risks of complete obliteration outweigh the benefit.[31] Untreated benign DAVFs and palliatively treated DAVFs carry a 2% and 1% risk of conversion to high-grade lesions, respectively.

Endovascular embolization
Endovascular treatment is considered the first-line treatment of higher grade DAVFs with cortical venous drainage that carry a 15% annual risk of neurologic defects and a 10.4% risk of mortality.[3,16,20,34,35] Endovascularly, the abnormal connection and proximal draining vein can be embolized transarterially or by transvenous catheterization. During transarterial embolization, distal arterial feeders are catheterized and liquid embolic

agents or coils are injected or inserted to occlude the draining vein while preserving the dural sinus (**Figs. 3–6**).[31,36] Transvenous embolization requires direct microcatheterization of the draining vein and embolization with a liquid embolic agent or coils (**Figs. 7–9**).[37] Transarterial embolization is usually conserved for special cases where the venous drainage is directed into a compartmentalized parallel channel within the dural sinus or draining venous pouch immediately proximal to a patent dural venous sinus.[31] When only feeding arteries are occluded and not the draining vein, collateral vessels usually develop and the DAVF can recur.[38] Sometimes a combined transvenous/transarterial approach is warranted and is achieved by transarterial injection of a liquid embolic while a transvenous balloon is inflated within the dural sinus to preserve patency.[39] The rate of radiological obliteration using endovascular therapy ranges from 69% to 95%.[31,40] The main concern with endovascular embolization is the risk of liquid embolic migration causing variable neurologic deficits based on the location of the feeding arteries.

Microsurgical treatment

Surgery is usually indicated after failure of endovascular embolization.[41] Historically, during surgery, the arterialized draining vein is ligated, arterial supply is disrupted, the involved dura is resected, and the diseased dural sinus is packed or skeletonized.[42,43] However, recent studies have shown that selective ligation of the arterialized vein without complete resection is more favorable with lower morbidity and long-term efficacy rates (**Figs. 10 and 11**).[44,45] The idea behind ligation of the arterialized vein is to occlude the fistula's sole venous outflow which indirectly obliterates shunting within the dura.[31] During the procedure, the adjunctive use of indocyanine green video angiography or Doppler ultrasound is encouraged to localize the arterialized vein and confirm complete obliteration. The rates of radiological obliteration following microsurgery range from 96% to 100%.[16,46–49] However, surgery carries risks with morbidity and mortality rates of 4.8% with selective ligation and 13% to 17% with complete resection.[16,47,48]

Stereotactic radiosurgery

Stereotactic radiosurgery (SRS) is reserved for DAVFs that are refractory to endovascular and surgical treatment and for patients with high-risk comorbidities.[50] Sometimes SRS is used as an adjuvant after subtotal embolization or surgical obliteration.[51] Because of the latency period of 1 to 3 years before DAVF obliteration, SRS is reserved for DAVF with benign angioarchitecture. Moreover, SRS is usually more effective for DAVFs located on major dural sinuses (transverse/sigmoid, torcula) compared to those with direct cortical drainage.[52] Using SRS, the radiological obliteration rate of DAVFs with and without cortical venous drainage is 56% and 75%, respectively.[52]

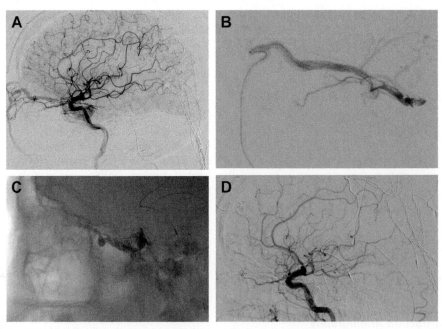

Fig. 9. (*A*) Angiography (lateral view) showing a cranial Barrow type D carotid cavernous fistula (CCF) with a prominent facial vein. (*B*) Microcatheter navigation from the superior orbital vein to the cavernous sinus. (*C*) X-ray showing Onyx cast. (*D*) Postoperative angiography (lateral view) showing complete occlusion of the CCF.

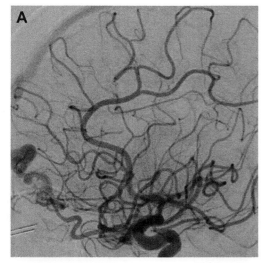

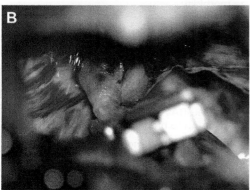

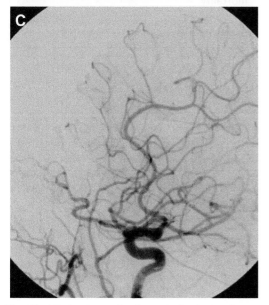

Fig. 10. (*A*) Angiography (lateral view) showing an ethmoidal dural arteriovenous fistula (DAVF). (*B*) Intraoperative figure showing clipping of the draining vein. (*C*). Postoperative angiography (lateral view) showing complete occlusion of the DAVF.

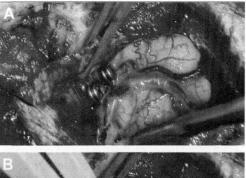

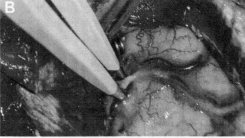

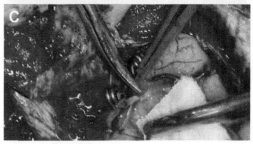

Fig. 11. Intracranial dural arteriovenous fistula (CDAVF) Borden type 3 with cortical venous drainage to the vein of Labbe. (*A*) Clipping of the fistulous connection to the vein of Labbe. (*B*) Cauterization of the veins using a bipolar cautery. (*C*) Disconnection of the veins.

Complications include post-radiation hemorrhage (1.2%), new/worsened neurologic deficits (1.3%), and mortality (0.3%).[52]

Combined therapy
Treatment of DAVFs should be patient-tailored and taking into consideration medical comorbidities, DAVF location, DAVF dimensions, DAVF classification, treatment success rates, and complication rates. Though embolization is the first-line treatment, using adjuvant therapy or staged treatment (embolization followed by resection) should be taken into consideration to optimize obliteration and minimize morbidity and mortality.

Spinal Dural Arteriovenous Fistulas

The 2 main treatment option for SDAVFs are endovascular therapy and open surgery. Unlike CDAVFs, the gold standard for SDAVFs is open surgery.[53] However, with recent advancements in endovascular techniques, it has been a matter of debate if endovascular embolization can comparable or higher rates of complete obliteration compared to open surgery.[54] To this date, several studies have shown that open surgery still provides higher rates of complete obliteration ranging between 96.6% and 99.3% compared to endovascular embolization (complete obliteration rate ranges between 46.6% and 72.2%%) (**Fig. 12**).[53,55] Moreover, there is still no consensus on which modality offers a better safety profile as some studies showed comparable morbidity rates while others showed lower morbidity rates with endovascular embolization.[53,55] Similar to CDAVFs, the main goal of SDAVF treatment is the obliteration of the arterialized vein. It is important to note that, during endovascular embolization, if the DAVF contains a common segmental artery that supplies both the fistula and the anterior or posterior spinal artery, surgical treatment might be preferred due to the high risk of morbidity in case of liquid embolic migration.[56] As for surgical treatment, correct localization of the fistula level is challenging and warrants intraoperative fluoroscopy or preoperative angiographic localization.[56]

SUMMARY

DAVFs are rare cerebrovascular lesions characterized by abnormal arteriovenous shunting within the dural leaflets. Significant variability exists regarding angioarchitecture and natural history. Early detection and diagnosis using the gold standard angiography is pivotal. Classification is essential and dictates treatment options. To this date, endovascular embolization is the first-line treatment of cranial DAVFs while surgical resection is the gold standard treatment option for SDAVFs. Combined therapy may be used in certain cases to provide maximal benefit and minimize morbidity.

CLINICS CARE POINTS

- Untreated benign DAVFs and conservatively managed DAVFs carry a 2 % and 1% risk of conversion to high-grade-lesions, respectively.
- Endovascular treatment is the first-line treatment of high grade DAVFs with cortical venous drainage and carries a 15% annual risk of neurologic defects and 10.4% risk of mortality.
- The rates of radiological obliteration following microsurgery range from 96% to 100%.

DISCLOSURE

Dr P. Jabbour is a consultant for Medtronic, MicroVention, Balt, and Cerus Endovascular. Dr S.I. Tjoumakaris is a consultant for MicroVention. Dr M.R. Gooch is a consultant for Stryker. Dr K. El Naamani has no personal, financial, or institutional interest in any of the drugs, materials, or devices described in this article.

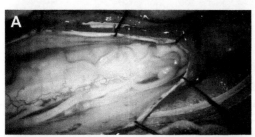
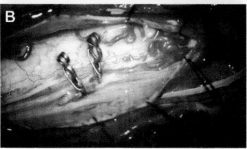
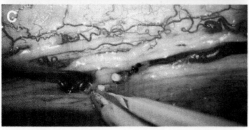

Fig. 12. (*A*) Intraoperative image showing a spinal dural arteriovenous fistula (SDAVF) highlighted using indocyanine green. (*B*) Clipping of the fistula. (*C*) Cauterization and disconnection of the arterialized vein.

REFERENCES

1. Elhammady MS, Ambekar S, Heros RC. Epidemiology, clinical presentation, diagnostic evaluation, and prognosis of cerebral dural arteriovenous fistulas. Handb Clin Neurol 2017;143:99–105.
2. Cognard C, Gobin YP, Pierot L, et al. Cerebral dural arteriovenous fistulas: clinical and angiographic correlation with a revised classification of venous drainage. Radiology 1995;194(3):671–80.

3. Zipfel GJ, Shah MN, Refai D, et al. Cranial dural arteriovenous fistulas: modification of angiographic classification scales based on new natural history data. Neurosurg Focus 2009;26(5):E14.

4. Martins C, Yasuda A, Campero A, et al. Microsurgical anatomy of the dural arteries. Neurosurgery 2005;56(2 Suppl):211–51 [discussion: 211–51].

5. Brown RD Jr, Wiebers DO, Nichols DA. Intracranial dural arteriovenous fistulae: angiographic predictors of intracranial hemorrhage and clinical outcome in nonsurgical patients. J Neurosurg 1994;81(4): 531–8.

6. Tsai LK, Liu HM, Jeng JS. Diagnosis and management of intracranial dural arteriovenous fistulas. Expert Rev Neurother 2016;16(3):307–18.

7. Hirono N, Yamadori A, Komiyama M. Dural arteriovenous fistula: a cause of hypoperfusion-induced intellectual impairment. Eur Neurol 1993;33(1):5–8.

8. Hurst RW, Bagley LJ, Galetta S, et al. Dementia resulting from dural arteriovenous fistulas: the pathologic findings of venous hypertensive encephalopathy. AJNR Am J Neuroradiol 1998;19(7): 1267–73.

9. Hasumi T, Fukushima T, Haisa T, et al. Focal dural arteriovenous fistula (DAVF) presenting with progressive cognitive impairment including amnesia and alexia. Intern Med 2007;46(16):1317–20.

10. Kendall BE, Logue V. Spinal epidural angiomatous malformations draining into intrathecal veins. Neuroradiology 1977;13(4):181–9.

11. Ali S, Cashen TA, Carroll TJ, et al. Time-resolved spinal MR angiography: initial clinical experience in the evaluation of spinal arteriovenous shunts. AJNR Am J Neuroradiol 2007;28(9):1806–10.

12. Schaat TJ, Salzman KL, Stevens EA. Sacral origin of a spinal dural arteriovenous fistula: case report and review. Spine 2002;27(8):893–7.

13. Geibprasert S, Pongpech S, Jiarakongmun P, et al. Cervical spine dural arteriovenous fistula presenting with congestive myelopathy of the conus. J Neurosurg Spine 2009;11(4):427–31.

14. Aminoff MJ, Barnard RO, Logue V. The pathophysiology of spinal vascular malformations. J Neurol Sci 1974;23(2):255–63.

15. Borden JA, Wu JK, Shucart WA. A proposed classification for spinal and cranial dural arteriovenous fistulous malformations and implications for treatment. J Neurosurg 1995;82(2):166–79.

16. Gross BA, Du R. The natural history of cerebral dural arteriovenous fistulae. Neurosurgery 2012;71(3): 594–602 [discussion: 602–3].

17. Shah MN, Botros JA, Pilgram TK, et al. Borden-Shucart Type I dural arteriovenous fistulas: clinical course including risk of conversion to higher-grade fistulas. J Neurosurg 2012;117(3):539–45.

18. Davies MA, Ter Brugge K, Willinsky R, et al. The natural history and management of intracranial dural arteriovenous fistulae. Part 2: aggressive lesions. Interv Neuroradiol 1997;3(4):303–11.

19. Bulters DO, Mathad N, Culliford D, et al. The natural history of cranial dural arteriovenous fistulae with cortical venous reflux–the significance of venous ectasia. Neurosurgery 2012;70(2):312–8 [discussion: 318–9].

20. van Dijk JM, terBrugge KG, Willinsky RA, et al. Clinical course of cranial dural arteriovenous fistulas with long-term persistent cortical venous reflux. Stroke 2002;33(5):1233–6.

21. van Rooij WJ, Sluzewski M, Beute GN. Intracranial dural fistulas with exclusive perimedullary drainage: the need for complete cerebral angiography for diagnosis and treatment planning. AJNR Am J Neuroradiol 2007;28(2):348–51.

22. Reynolds MR, Lanzino G, Zipfel GJ. Intracranial Dural Arteriovenous Fistulae. Stroke 2017;48(5): 1424–31.

23. Daniels DJ, Vellimana AK, Zipfel GJ, et al. Intracranial hemorrhage from dural arteriovenous fistulas: clinical features and outcome. Neurosurg Focus 2013;34(5):E15.

24. Holekamp TF, Mollman ME, Murphy RK, et al. Dural arteriovenous fistula-induced thalamic dementia: report of 4 cases. J Neurosurg 2016;124(6):1752–65.

25. Letourneau-Guillon L, Cruz JP, Krings T. CT and MR imaging of non-cavernous cranial dural arteriovenous fistulas: Findings associated with cortical venous reflux. Eur J Radiol 2015;84(8):1555–63.

26. Sato K, Shimizu H, Fujimura M, et al. Compromise of brain tissue caused by cortical venous reflux of intracranial dural arteriovenous fistulas: assessment with diffusion-weighted magnetic resonance imaging. Stroke 2011;42(4):998–1003.

27. Noguchi K, Kubo M, Kuwayama N, et al. Intracranial dural arteriovenous fistulas with retrograde cortical venous drainage: assessment with cerebral blood volume by dynamic susceptibility contrast magnetic resonance imaging. AJNR Am J Neuroradiol 2006; 27(6):1252–6.

28. Naamani KE, Abbas R, Tartaglino L, et al. The Accuracy of the TRICKS MRI in Diagnosing and Localizing a Spinal Dural Arteriovenous Fistula: A Feasibility Study. World Neurosurg 2022;158: e592–7.

29. Willinsky R, Goyal M, terBrugge K, et al. Tortuous, engorged pial veins in intracranial dural arteriovenous fistulas: correlations with presentation, location, and MR findings in 122 patients. AJNR Am J Neuroradiol 1999;20(6):1031–6.

30. Willinsky R, Lasjaunias P, Terbrugge K, et al. Angiography in the investigation of spinal dural arteriovenous fistula. A protocol with application of the venous phase. Neuroradiology 1990;32(2):114–6.

31. Oushy S, Borg N, Lanzino G. Contemporary Management of Cranial Dural Arteriovenous Fistulas. World Neurosurg 2022;159:288–97.

32. Baharvahdat H, Ooi YC, Kim WJ, et al. Updates in the management of cranial dural arteriovenous fistula. Stroke Vasc Neurol 2020;5(1):50–8.

33. Samaniego EA, Roa JA, Hayakawa M, et al. Dural arteriovenous fistulas without cortical venous drainage: presentation, treatment, and outcomes. J Neurosurg 2022;136(4):942–50.

34. Strom RG, Botros JA, Refai D, et al. Cranial dural arteriovenous fistulae: asymptomatic cortical venous drainage portends less aggressive clinical course. Neurosurgery 2009;64(2):241–7 [discussion: 247–8].

35. Duffau H, Lopes M, Janosevic V, et al. Early rebleeding from intracranial dural arteriovenous fistulas: report of 20 cases and review of the literature. J Neurosurg 1999;90(1):78–84.

36. Chandra RV, Leslie-Mazwi TM, Mehta BP, et al. Transarterial onyx embolization of cranial dural arteriovenous fistulas: long-term follow-up. AJNR Am J Neuroradiol 2014;35(9):1793–7.

37. Zhang S, Wang J, Liu D, et al. Embolization of Cavernous Sinus Dural Arteriovenous Fistula (CSDAVF) via transvenous approaches: Practice, experience summary and literature review. J Clin Neurosci 2021;89:283–91.

38. Mullan S. Reflections upon the nature and management of intracranial and intraspinal vascular malformations and fistulae. J Neurosurg 1994;80(4):606–16.

39. Signorelli F, Della Pepa GM, Sabatino G, et al. Diagnosis and management of dural arteriovenous fistulas: a 10 years single-center experience. Clin Neurol Neurosurg 2015;128:123–9.

40. Oh JS, Yoon SM, Oh HJ, et al. Endovascular Treatment of Dural Arteriovenous Fistulas: Single Center Experience. J Korean Neurosurg Soc 2016;59(1):17–25.

41. Lawton MT, Chun J, Wilson CB, et al. Ethmoidal dural arteriovenous fistulae: an assessment of surgical and endovascular management. Neurosurgery 1999;45(4):805–10 [discussion: 810–1].

42. Youssef PP, Schuette AJ, Cawley CM, et al. Advances in surgical approaches to dural fistulas. Neurosurgery 2014;74(Suppl 1):S32–41.

43. Thompson BG, Doppman JL, Oldfield EH. Treatment of cranial dural arteriovenous fistulae by interruption of leptomeningeal venous drainage. J Neurosurg 1994;80(4):617–23.

44. van Dijk JM, TerBrugge KG, Willinsky RA, et al. Selective disconnection of cortical venous reflux as treatment for cranial dural arteriovenous fistulas. J Neurosurg 2004;101(1):31–5.

45. Collice M, D'Aliberti G, Talamonti G, et al. Surgical interruption of leptomeningeal drainage as treatment for intracranial dural arteriovenous fistulas without dural sinus drainage. J Neurosurg 1996;84(5):810–7.

46. Al-Mahfoudh R, Kirollos R, Mitchell P, et al. Surgical disconnection of the cortical venous reflux for high-grade intracranial dural arteriovenous fistulas. World Neurosurg 2015;83(4):652–6.

47. Wachter D, Hans F, Psychogios MN, et al. Microsurgery can cure most intracranial dural arteriovenous fistulae of the sinus and non-sinus type. Neurosurg Rev 2011;34(3):337–45 [discussion: 345].

48. Kakarla UK, Deshmukh VR, Zabramski JM, et al. Surgical treatment of high-risk intracranial dural arteriovenous fistulae: clinical outcomes and avoidance of complications. Neurosurgery 2007;61(3):447–57 [discussion: 457–9].

49. Liu JK, Dogan A, Ellegala DB, et al. The role of surgery for high-grade intracranial dural arteriovenous fistulas: importance of obliteration of venous outflow. J Neurosurg 2009;110(5):913–20.

50. Loumiotis I, Lanzino G, Daniels D, et al. Radiosurgery for intracranial dural arteriovenous fistulas (DAVFs): a review. Neurosurg Rev 2011;34(3):305–15 [discussion: 315].

51. Friedman JA, Pollock BE, Nichols DA, et al. Results of combined stereotactic radiosurgery and transarterial embolization for dural arteriovenous fistulas of the transverse and sigmoid sinuses. J Neurosurg 2001;94(6):886–91.

52. Chen CJ, Lee CC, Ding D, et al. Stereotactic radiosurgery for intracranial dural arteriovenous fistulas: a systematic review. J Neurosurg 2015;122(2):353–62.

53. Takai K, Endo T, Yasuhara T, et al. Neurosurgical versus endovascular treatment of spinal dural arteriovenous fistulas: a multicenter study of 195 patients. J Neurosurg Spine 2020;34(3):514–21.

54. Steinmetz MP, Chow MM, Krishnaney AA, et al. Outcome after the treatment of spinal dural arteriovenous fistulae: a contemporary single-institution series and meta-analysis. Neurosurgery 2004;55(1):77–87 [discussion: 87–8].

55. Goyal A, Cesare J, Lu VM, et al. Outcomes following surgical versus endovascular treatment of spinal dural arteriovenous fistula: a systematic review and meta-analysis. J Neurol Neurosurg Psychiatry 2019;90(10):1139–46.

56. Dehdashti AR, Da Costa LB, terBrugge KG, et al. Overview of the current role of endovascular and surgical treatment in spinal dural arteriovenous fistulas. Neurosurg Focus 2009;26(1):E8.

Cerebral Venous Sinus Thrombosis

Vincent N. Nguyen, MD, Alexandra N. Demetriou, MA, Jonathan Dallas, MD, William J. Mack, MD, MBA*

KEYWORDS

- Cerebral • Venous sinus • Cortical vein • Thrombectomy • Endovascular • Anticoagulation • Stroke
- Headache

KEY POINTS

- Cerebral venous sinus thrombosis (CVST) is a rare stroke involving blood clot formation in the dural venous sinuses, predominantly affecting younger individuals, especially women.
- Historically, CVST was associated with high mortality rates, but advancements in neuroimaging have improved diagnosis and prognosis, with mortality rates less than 10%.
- Risk factors and predisposing conditions, including prothrombotic conditions, pregnancy, cancer, autoimmune diseases, systemic disorders, infections, and iatrogenic causes, contribute to CVST development.
- Pathophysiology of CVST involves venous stasis, endothelial damage, and hypercoagulability, leading to thrombus formation, venous hypertension, cerebral ischemia, and potential hemorrhagic conversion.
- Clinical presentation varies but often includes headaches, increased intracranial pressure, seizures, and focal neurologic deficits. Prompt diagnosis via CT or MR venography is essential for effective management. Treatment involves anticoagulation, and endovascular therapies may be considered in refractory cases. The prognosis is generally favorable with timely intervention.

INTRODUCTION
Definition of Cerebral Venous Sinus Thrombosis

Cerebral venous sinus thrombosis (CVST) is a rare type of stroke characterized by the formation of blood clots within the dural venous sinuses, which are large venous conduits that are located between the two layers of the dura mater and are responsible for draining blood from the brain and returning it to the systemic circulation.[1] More specifically, cortical venous thrombosis refers to the blockage of veins on the brain's cortical surface. Cerebral venous thrombosis (CVT) encompasses both dural and cortical vein occlusions.[2] CVST is a relatively uncommon stroke subtype, estimated to be between 0.5% and 1% of all stroke cases, and predominantly affects younger individuals.[2]

Historical Perspective

CVST was first recognized in the early nineteenth century as an infectious ailment that tends to affect the superior sagittal sinus. This often led to bilateral or alternating focal deficits, seizures, and coma, resulting in a high mortality rate. In 1825, Ribes provided a comprehensive account of a 45 year old man's bout with CVST that ended in his demise.[3] For 6 months, the patient endured debilitating symptoms, including severe headaches, epileptic seizures, and episodes of delirium. A postmortem examination revealed thrombus in the superior sagittal sinus, the left transverse sinus, and a left parietal cortical vein.

CVST was typically diagnosed postmortem during this early period and was associated with hemorrhagic lesions. However, over the past 25 years,

Department of Neurosurgery, University of Southern California, 1520 San Pablo Street, Suite 3800, Los Angeles, CA 90033, USA
* Corresponding author.
E-mail address: William.Mack@med.usc.edu

Neurosurg Clin N Am 35 (2024) 343–353
https://doi.org/10.1016/j.nec.2024.02.006
1042-3680/24/© 2024 Elsevier Inc. All rights reserved.

the widespread adoption of neuroimaging techniques has enabled more accurate and timely diagnosis. CVST is now generally recognized as a noninfectious disorder with diverse clinical manifestations and, more importantly, a favorable prognosis, with mortality rates well below 10%.[4]

Epidemiology of Cerebral Venous Sinus Thrombosis

In the 1970s, a study of 182 consecutive autopsies found that CVST incidence was 9.3%.[5] Several early investigations have reported the incidence to be between 2 and 5 cases per million individuals per year, with an increased incidence in the most recent population-based studies ranging from 12 to 15 per million.[6–8] CVST more often affects young adults with a mean age of 35 years and is more typical in women due to sex-specific risk factors.[9] The annual incidence of CVST in children is roughly 7 cases per million, affecting neonates more commonly than children.[9]

DISCUSSION
Overview of Risk Factors and Predisposing Conditions for Cerebral Venous Sinus Thrombosis

CVST arises from a complex interplay of various risk factors. These factors can be broadly categorized into acquired risks, such as surgery, trauma, or pregnancy, and genetic predispositions, known as inherited thrombophilia.[2]

Prothrombotic conditions: The most extensively studied CVST risk factors fall under the umbrella of prothrombotic conditions. In the ISCVT study, 34% of patients displayed either inherited or acquired prothrombotic conditions, which primarily include[2]

- Antithrombin III, protein C, and protein S deficiency
- Antiphospholipid and anticardiolipin antibodies
- Factor V Leiden gene mutation and resistance to activated protein C
- Prothrombin G20210A mutation
- Hyperhomocysteinemia

Pregnancy, puerperium, and the usage of oral contraceptives create temporary prothrombotic states, contributing to CVST risk.[2] *Cancer* is linked to a fraction of CVST cases, with potential mechanisms including tumor compression, sinus invasion, and hypercoagulable state associated with malignancies. Chemotherapy and hormonal agents used in cancer treatment may also contribute.

Autoimmune disease: Neuro-Behçet syndrome and systemic lupus erythematosus (SLE) are 2 autoimmune conditions associated with CVST. Neuro-Behçet syndrome occurs in 5% to 10% of cases of Behçet disease and can take either an intra-axial or extra-axial form. Its extra-axial form, present in approximately 10% to 20% of individuals, may lead to CVST.[10] SLE is another rare cause of CVST. Neurologic involvement occurs in 3% to 20% of patients with SLE, and the development of CVST is strongly correlated with the presence of antiphospholipid antibodies and lupus anticoagulant.[11]

Systemic disorders: Hyperthyroidism is generally considered to have a stronger association with CVST than hypothyroidism. Thyroid hormone is proposed to increase circulating clotting factors, fibrinogen, von Willebrand factor, and plasminogen activator inhibitor-1, increasing the likelihood of thrombus formation.[12]

Other uncommon risk factors include infections, paroxysmal nocturnal hemoglobinuria, and iron-deficiency anemia. These factors account for a minority of CVST cases and are less common in adults.

Iatrogenic causes of venous thrombosis have also been reported, resulting from various skull base neurosurgical approaches, direct sinus injury, or intracranial hypotension due to cerebrospinal fluid (CSF) leakage after lumbar puncture or spinal anesthesia.

Pathophysiology of Cerebral Venous Sinus Thrombosis

Venous stasis, endothelial damage, and hypercoagulability, collectively known as Virchow's triad, result in an imbalance between prothrombotic and fibrinolytic processes.[13] Proinflammatory states such as trauma or infection lead to cytokine production and increased coagulation cascade activation.[14] Trauma or neurosurgical procedures can damage venous endothelium and create a nidus upon which thrombosis may occur. Underlying disorders contributing to platelet dysfunction or imbalances between procoagulant and anticoagulant molecules may also promote thrombus formation.

CVST causes venous hypertension and blood vessel dilation, leading to brain edema. Decreased venous outflow reduces capillary perfusion pressure, and reduced blood flow causes local cerebral ischemia. Impaired oxygen delivery needed for Na/K ATPases results in an influx of water and subsequent cell death, which is characteristic of cytotoxic edema, more so than the extracellular fluid shifts seen in vasogenic edema. Over time, venous hypertension can tear veins, resulting in subarachnoid and intraparenchymal hemorrhages.[15]

Clinical Presentation

The clinical presentation of CVST is diverse and can vary depending on the underlying cause, the duration of the disease, and the specific veins and sinuses affected. Acute cases of CVST are often linked to infectious or obstetric causes, while subacute and chronic cases are more commonly associated with inflammatory disorders.[16]

In most CVST cases, headache is the most frequently reported initial symptom, occurring in 74% to 90% of patients.[1] A study of 200 CVST patients found 136 experienced headaches lasting 1 to 3 days at diagnosis.[17] These headaches may resemble migraines but may be exacerbated by activities like coughing or head movements. Rarely, they can manifest as "thunderclap" headaches, characteristic of acute CVST but more classically associated with subarachnoid hemorrhage.[18] Elevated intracranial pressure (ICP) can lead to nausea, vomiting, vertigo, dizziness, and visual disturbances, with or without papilledema.

Focal neurologic deficits may develop hours or days after the headache in about half of CVST patients. Common syndromes include leg weakness or hemiparesis due to infarction in the frontoparietal regions surrounding the vein of Trolard. Aphasia and confusion may result from infarction around the vein of Labbé in the temporal lobe. Sigmoid sinus involvement can cause mastoid pain and, rarely, lower cranial neuropathies. Encephalopathy or coma may occur, mainly due to multiple sinus or deep venous occlusions, sometimes accompanied by increased ICP. These deficits may fluctuate and are often reversible but do not align with typical arterial stroke territories.[13] Seizures occur in up to 40% of patients within a week following thrombosis, with varying rates of potentially treatment-refractory status epilepticus.[13,19]

Chronic CVST can cause long-standing headaches with papilledema, tinnitus, ocular palsy, and exophthalmos, which may lead to intracranial hypertension and dural arteriovenous fistulae.[4,20,21]

Cavernous sinus thrombosis manifests as a regional syndrome with periorbital and forehead pain, ocular chemosis, and cranial nerve palsies affecting the third, fourth, and sixth cranial nerves, as well as the ophthalmic and maxillary divisions of the fifth cranial nerve as they pass through the cavernous sinus. Brainstem and cerebellar signs may occur if thrombosis extends from the cavernous to the petrosal sinuses.[1,22]

Diagnostic Approaches and Imaging Modalities

Computerized tomography (CT) of the head without contrast is often the first imaging modality completed in the diagnostic workup (**Fig. 1**). On CT, CVST appears as a hyperdense signal in the vessel lumen in the acute phase and then progresses to appearing isodense and finally hypodense after 1 week.[9] Some specific signs include the "dense triangle" in the setting of superior sagittal sinus thrombosis, the "dense cord" seen in cortical or deep venous thrombosis,[9] or "cashew nut" for juxtacortical hemorrhages, which are small (<20 mm), concave-shaped and located just below the cortex exclusively in the white matter.[23] Nevertheless, initial noncontrast head CT may appear normal in 25% to 30% of patients.[24] MRI confers additional sensitivity to identify thromboses at different time points along the disease course and achieve better resolution of potential findings, including hemorrhagic and infarcted regions, parenchymal edema, and sulcal effacement (**Fig. 2**).[2,25] CT or MRI with contrast may reveal an "empty delta" sign, consisting of a hypodense triangle surrounded by enhancement that indicates superior sagittal sinus thrombosis.[25,26]

CT venography (CTV) and MR venography (MRV), preferably with contrast, are considered the optimal imaging modalities for CVST and should be performed in all suspected cases (**Fig. 3**). MRV or CTV should demonstrate one or more filling defects in the setting of CVST. CTV is performed more rapidly, while MRV provides the benefits of enhanced resolution and avoids radiation exposure. Asymmetries of the sigmoid plate notch on CT can reliably differentiate a congenitally atretic sinus from thrombosis in cases with absent MRV signals.[27] If MRV and CTV are inconclusive, formal catheter-based cerebral angiography may be performed to confirm CVST (**Fig. 4**).[9] The normal cerebral venous system typically opacifies in 7 to 8 seconds on angiography. One can suspect acute thrombosis if cerebral veins or sinuses do not opacify within this time frame.[2]

Although no laboratory test confirms the diagnosis of CVST, routine laboratory studies and measurement of D-dimer are still typically performed in the diagnostic workup. Screening may be performed to identify underlying disorders contributing to a hypercoagulable state, particularly in patients with a high pretest probability of severe thrombophilia.[2] Lumbar puncture is typically only indicated to rule out meningitis if suspected.[2]

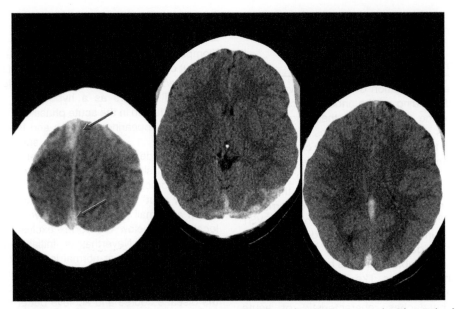

Fig. 1. A patient in her 20s with migraines on oral contraceptive medications presented with a 5 day history of worsening headaches. This progressed to nausea, vomiting, left-sided weakness, and then obtundation. She was intubated and transferred to our institution. On examination, she was not following commands and only localizing to pain. CT scan demonstrated pan venous sinus occlusion, as evidenced by the hyperdensities in the superior sagittal sinus (SSS), right parietal cortical vein, left transverse/sigmoid sinuses, and straight sinus (*red arrows*).

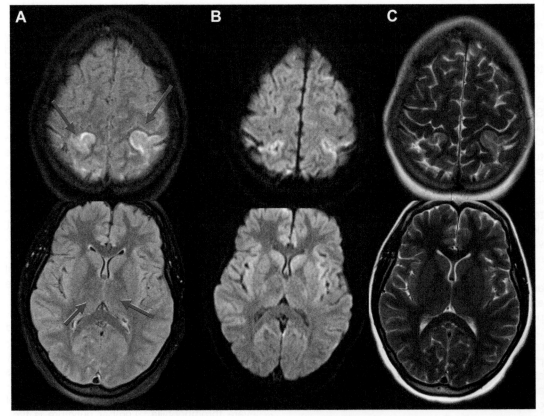

Fig. 2. MRI sequences (*A*) FLAIR, (*B*) DWI, and (*C*) T2 demonstrate biparietal ischemia with marked hyperintensities, with no significant thalamic ischemia despite the deep venous involvement. *Top red arrows* indicate the FLAIR ischemic changes in the biparietal lobes. *Bottom red arrows* indicate the lack of ischemic changes in the bilateral thalami.

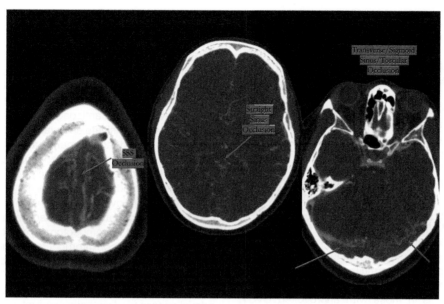

Fig. 3. CTV demonstrates multiple venous sinus occlusions (*red arrows*) with a lack of contrast opacification of the entirety of the SSS, the straight sinus/vein of Galen, and the bilateral transverse sinuses.

Medical Management and Treatment Options

Treatment Guidelines from the American Heart Association (AHA) and the European Stroke Organization emphasize the importance of promptly initiating anticoagulation upon diagnosing CVST to prevent thrombus propagation and facilitate recanalization.[2,28] Sinus recanalization is closely linked to functional recovery, with a 3.3 fold increase in the odds of favorable outcome (modified rankin scale [mRS] 0–1), while the lack of venous recanalization is associated with poorer outcomes.[29]

After initiating anticoagulation therapy, the recanalization rate has been reported to range from 47% to 100%; most cases recanalize within the initial few months post-treatment for CVST, though recanalization may take up to 1 year.[29]

The use of heparin and anticoagulation for CVST treatment has long been debated due to concerns over exacerbating intracerebral hemorrhage (ICH). However, in the 1990s, 2 randomized controlled trials involving 79 patients provided compelling evidence in favor of anticoagulation. These studies demonstrated decreased mortality rates and improved functional outcomes in patients receiving anticoagulation, even in cases with pre-existing ICH.[30,31]

Seeking formal consultation with an anticoagulation management expert may be judicious, especially in cases with significant contraindications to full anticoagulation, such as other major recent hemorrhages. Exploring the possibility of low-intensity anticoagulation regimens may be advantageous in these circumstances.[2]

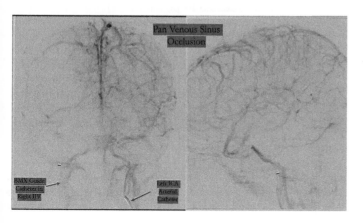

Fig. 4. Formal catheter angiography was performed via a transradial arterial approach using a 5 Fr Simmons catheter placed in the left internal carotid artery and a transfemoral venous approach using an 8 Fr Guide catheter placed in the right internal jugular vein.

Anticoagulant considerations

Most available data on anticoagulation for CVST in the acute phase support using unfractionated heparin (UFH) or low-molecular-weight heparin (LMWH). Meta-analyses and guidelines on the treatment of venous thromboembolism (VTE), including deep vein thrombosis, pulmonary embolism (PE), and CVST, suggest a decreased risk of major bleeding events, including ICHs, with LMWH compared to UFH with moderate quality evidence.[2,28,32]

After initiating anticoagulation with LMWH or UFH, one must bridge to oral anticoagulation with a vitamin K antagonist (VKA) to promote recanalization and prevent CVST recurrence or other venous thromboembolic events. The AHA guidelines recommend bridging to a VKA with a target international normalized ratio of 2 to 3 for 3 to 6 months in patients with provoked CVST, 6 to 12 months in those with unprovoked CVST, and indefinite anticoagulation in patients with recurrent CVST, VTE after CVST, or those with severe thrombophilia experiencing their first CVST event.[2]

With the advent of direct oral anticoagulants (DOACs), data continue to emerge regarding their benefits compared to VKAs. One randomized trial compared patients with CVST treated with warfarin or dabigatran after initial systemic anticoagulation with intravenous (IV) heparin. Warfarin and dabigatran showed similar bleeding risks and comparable recanalization rates, with no recurrent VTE events in either group.[33] Recent meta-analyses have demonstrated comparable efficacy and safety between the 2 agents regarding risks of recurrent VTE, major hemorrhage, ICH, death, and complete venous recanalization.[34]

Endovascular Management

While most patients with CVST recover with anticoagulation therapy alone, approximately 20% may continue to deteriorate despite adequate anticoagulation.[2,28,35] Endovascular treatment options may aid in rapidly reducing thrombus burden, promoting recanalization, and alleviating venous congestion. However, much of the available data on endovascular treatments for CVST are derived from retrospective case reports and case series and are thus prone to bias.[36] A recent systematic review of 17 retrospective studies with 235 patients found complete radiographic resolution of CVST in 69% of patients, with 34.7% neurologically intact at follow-up (0.5–3.5 years) and a 14.3% mortality rate.[37] CVST recurred in only 1.2% of cases; new or worsening ICH occurred in 8.7%. The only multicenter randomized controlled trial studying systemic anticoagulation with or without endovascular therapy was stopped prematurely for futility after the first interim analysis.[38]

The subgroups that may benefit (refractory intracranial hypertension, progressive venous infarction, or hematoma expansion) remain ill-defined. Additionally, there are no well-established criteria for determining when anticoagulation therapy has failed and when to initiate endovascular treatment. Given the limited and largely case-based evidence, the AHA suggests that endovascular management be considered if clinical deterioration occurs during medical management.[2]

Numerous endovascular techniques exist for CVST, including catheter-directed thrombolysis, direct aspiration thrombectomy, stent-retriever thrombectomy, balloon thrombectomy, and balloon angioplasty with stenting. There are insufficient data to favor one technique over another.[37,39,40] Successful application of these approaches requires arterial access for diagnostic cerebral angiography and venous access for the intervention.

CATHETER-DIRECTED THROMBOLYSIS

Numerous reports have described using various thrombolytic agents, including urokinase, streptokinase, and tissue plasminogen activator (alteplase). For example, a microcatheter infusion of intra-sinus alteplase can be administered at 1 to 2 mg/hour, with repeat angiography performed at 12 to 24 hours to assess the response to thrombolysis and guide treatment decisions.[40] Catheter-directed thrombolysis has also been effectively used as an adjunct in multimodality endovascular treatment.[40,41] However, a systematic review reported new ICH in 17% of patients after thrombolysis, with 5% experiencing clinical deterioration.[42]

DIRECT ASPIRATION THROMBECTOMY

Large-bore distal aspiration catheters, initially designed for intra-arterial thrombectomies, have been adapted to perform thrombus aspiration in CVST. The largest aspiration catheters (2–3 mm) are still much smaller than the average diameter of the superior sagittal sinus (10 mm); thus, they are imperfect for direct aspiration and often cause significant blood loss.[20] The primary treatment of CVST with direct aspiration alone may expedite venous sinus recanalization without thrombolytics while achieving similar recanalization rates and favorable outcomes.

STENT-RETRIEVER THROMBECTOMY

Stent-retriever thrombectomy devices have also been adapted effectively for CVST treatment alone or in conjunction with catheter-directed thrombolysis or aspiration. They can also serve as anchors to assist with navigating aspiration catheters further distally within the venous sinuses (**Fig. 5**).[20,40,41]

BALLOON THROMBECTOMY

Another mechanical thrombectomy technique involves using a balloon that is advanced past the thrombus site, inflated and then retracted toward an aspiration catheter to macerate and dislodge the thrombus. Fogarty 3 or 4 French or other lower profile compliant or semicompliant neurovascular balloon catheters have been used successfully, sometimes combined with thrombolytic therapy to prevent PE.[20]

BALLOON VENOPLASTY AND STENTING

Some cases of refractory CVST have been managed with balloon venoplasty and stent placement with postoperative anticoagulation and antiplatelet therapy. This approach has shown promise in achieving persistent recanalization of the treated venous sinuses.[40]

Open Surgical Management

Open surgical venous sinus thrombectomy
Open sinus thrombectomy has been historically performed in cases of severe, refractory CVST that do not respond to anticoagulation therapy with significant improvements in functional outcomes.[2,43] The increasing use and efficacy of endovascular approaches may further diminish the role of open thrombectomy.

Decompressive craniectomy
CVST patients with severe intracranial hypertension, sinus thrombosis extension, or mass lesions such as hemorrhagic venous infarcts may progress to transtentorial herniation.[44] Decompressive craniectomy, although not a direct treatment for sinus

thrombosis, can be a life-saving procedure that offers the possibility of good functional outcomes. Several series have reported 57% to 77% of patients achieving a modified Rankin scale score of 0 to 2 at 6 to 12 month follow-up following decompressive craniectomy.[45,46] Decompressive surgery may be particularly beneficial if performed within 12 hours of admission or in patients less than 40 years.[46] The timing of resuming systemic anticoagulation after craniectomy remains poorly understood, with some recommendations suggesting initiation of heparin 6 to 24 hours after surgery.[46,47]

Prognosis and Potential Complications

If identified and treated promptly, CVST prognosis is typically good (**Figs. 6** and **7**). Approximately 80% of patients recover completely from their initial event, and only 2% experience recurrence in the first 16 months thereafter.[35] The following are potential complications associated with CVST:

Seizures
Early seizure onset during the acute phase of CVST presentation is associated with poorer prognosis during the first month of recovery.[48] The liberal use of antiepileptics for symptomatic seizures, particularly with parenchymal lesions, is recommended, while prophylactic antiepileptics are not.[2]

Hydrocephalus
CVST can hinder the normal functioning of arachnoid granulations in absorbing CSF, leading to communicating hydrocephalus in 4% to 6% of cases.[15] Obstructive hydrocephalus may occur due to intraventricular hemorrhage from deep venous infarction. Temporary or permanent CSF diversion may be required for treatment.

Intracranial hypertension
Forty percent of patients with CVST may manifest isolated intracranial hypertension with symptoms such as papilledema or third and sixth nerve

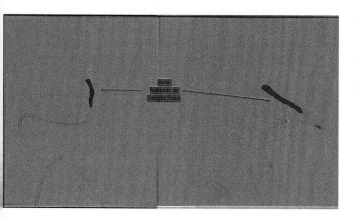

Fig. 5. Given the extensive venous sinus occlusion and her deteriorating neurologic examination, multiple aspiration attempts were performed in conjunction with deploying a 6 × 40 mm stent-retriever device as an anchor in the straight sinus and SSS.

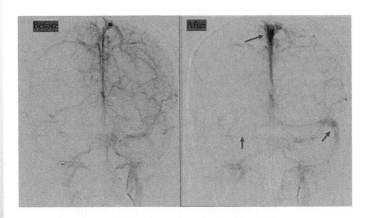

Fig. 6. Anterior-posterior angiography in the venous phase demonstrates significant venous congestion and no filling of the occluded venous sinuses before endovascular thrombectomy. Postintervention, there is restoration of flow in the SSS and bilateral transverse/sigmoid sinuses (*red arrows*) and resolution of the cortical venous congestion.

palsies.[49] Prolonged papilledema can lead to permanent blindness unless the elevated ICP is addressed through CSF diversion. Acetazolamide, a carbonic anhydrase inhibitor, can address intracranial hypertension in CVST as a mild diuretic and reduce CSF production.[13,19] Optic nerve sheath fenestration has also been used to manage papilledema and vision loss.[50]

Special Considerations

Cerebral venous sinus thrombosis in pediatric populations

CVST in children is uncommon, with an estimated incidence rate of 7 per million children annually.[9] Neonates are more frequently affected than older children. In children, otitis media and mastoiditis are among the most common triggers of CVST. Infantile CVST may be associated with obstetric conditions such as premature rupture of membranes, maternal hypertensive disorders, maternal infections, and gestational diabetes.

The clinical presentation of CVST in children is generally more nonspecific than in adults. Children are more likely to present with seizures, and neurologic deficits in children are often more generalized than focal.[51] Diagnostic modalities in children are similar to those in adults. In neonates, ultrasonography of the venous vasculature may be performed through patent fontanelles or on prenatal ultrasound. Gestational CVSTs may spontaneously resolve, though the condition can be mistaken for an intracranial tumor on imaging and may prompt parents to terminate pregnancy therapeutically. Imaging such as lesions with color Doppler sonography is necessary to diagnose accurately and counsel parents accordingly.[52]

Conservative management may be sufficient for pediatric CVST; in all patients, care should be taken to correct dehydration and address underlying disorders.[53] UFH and LMWH are the most commonly used anticoagulants in the acute phase and have been demonstrated to be safe and effective in children. Transition to long-term anticoagulation needs to be better defined in the pediatric population. However, 3 to 6 months is commonly recommended in children, whereas shorter period of 6 weeks to 3 months is used in neonates.

The mortality rate for pediatric CVST is 10%, except for neonates, for whom mortality is estimated at 25% to 50%.[53] Anywhere from 20% to

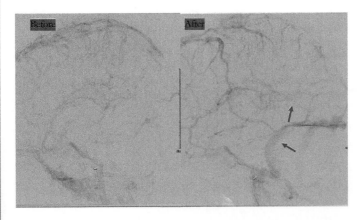

Fig. 7. Lateral angiography in the venous phase demonstrates the filling of the deep venous structures (vein of Galen, straight sinus: *red arrows*) and sigmoid sinuses. She made a remarkable recovery and was discharged postoperative day 7, neurologically intact. She was transitioned from a full-dose heparin drip to apixaban (factor Xa inhibitor), and her hypercoagulable workup was negative.

70% of patients suffer long-term neurologic deficits, including learning disabilities, sixth nerve palsy, motor and sensory impairments, visual disturbances, and headaches.[53] Surveillance MRV or CTV is typically performed at 3, 6, and 12 month intervals following resolution of the acute phase to monitor for recurrence or hydrocephalus.[53]

Cerebral venous sinus thrombosis and the link to COVID-19

COVID-19 infection has an established association with thrombotic events, likely due to increased cytokine release and endothelial damage secondary to angiotensin-converting-enzyme 2 (ACE2) receptor binding by the virus.[54] This association with hypercoagulability is shared with other respiratory viruses of the twenty-first century, including influenza A virus H1N1 subtype, Middle East respiratory syndrome, and severe acute respiratory syndrome.[55] The incidence of CVST secondary to COVID-19 infection is estimated to be 231 per million person-years.[56] Nonspecific symptoms such as headaches may be attributed to viral infection, leading to delays in diagnosis.

CVST has been observed following COVID-19 vaccination in the context of vaccine-induced immune thrombotic thrombocytopenia (VITT) and is associated with in anti-PF4 antibodies.[57] VITT occurs more frequently with DNA-based adenoviral vector COVID-19 vaccines.[58] CVST may occur in as many as half of patients who develop VITT,[59] and mortality rates are estimated at 39% to 64%, making CVST one of the most concerning, albeit rare, complications following COVID-19 vaccination.[60,61]

Management of CVST in the setting of VITT differs from general CVST management. Given the presumed pathophysiologic relationship to heparin-induced thrombocytopenia, DOACs or direct thrombin inhibitors are preferred.[62] Additionally, intravenous immune globulin and glucocorticoids aid in normalizing platelet counts.

SUMMARY

CVST is a rare type of stroke characterized by blood clot formation in the dural venous sinuses. Its incidence is increasing and tends to affect younger female individuals and patients with underlying prothrombotic conditions. The clinical presentation of CVST is diverse, with symptoms including headaches, increased ICP, seizures, and neurologic deficits. CTV and MRV can confirm the diagnosis. Anticoagulation remains the mainstay of therapy, even with ICH. Endovascular therapies are reserved for cases refractory to traditional medical management. The prognosis for most patients is favorable with timely diagnosis and management of complications.

CLINICS CARE POINTS

- Maintain a high index of suspicion for CVST, especially in patients presenting with severe headaches, neurologic deficits, seizures, or risk factors such as prothrombotic conditions, recent surgery, or pregnancy.

- Head CT scans are an effective initial imaging modality. However, be aware that they may appear normal in some cases. MRV or CTV can provide a definitive diagnosis.

- Initiate anticoagulation therapy promptly upon diagnosis, with UFH or LMWH as first-line options, and bridge to oral anticoagulation with a VKA for long-term management.

- Evaluate for underlying prothrombotic conditions, including inherited or acquired factors such as antithrombin III, protein C, protein S deficiency, factor V Leiden mutation, and antiphospholipid antibodies, as they may guide treatment decisions and prognosis.

- Consider endovascular treatments for patients with severe or refractory CVST. Reserve decompressive craniectomy for patients with severe intracranial hypertension or mass lesions at risk for transtentorial herniation.

DISCLOSURE

The authors have no financial or industry connections relevant to the contents of this article.

REFERENCES

1. Ropper AH, Klein JP. Cerebral Venous Thrombosis. N Engl J Med 2021;385(1):59–64.
2. Saposnik G, Barinagarrementeria F, Brown RD Jr, et al. Diagnosis and management of cerebral venous thrombosis: a statement for healthcare professionals from the American Heart Association/American Stroke Association. Stroke 2011;42(4):1158–92.
3. Ribes F. Exposé succinct des recherches faites sur la phlébite. Paris, France: Gueffier; 1825.
4. Bousser MG, Ferro JM. Cerebral venous thrombosis: an update. Lancet Neurol 2007;6(2):162–70.
5. Towbin A. The syndrome of latent cerebral venous thrombosis: its frequency and relation to age and congestive heart failure. Stroke 1973;4(3):419–30.
6. Coutinho JM, Zuurbier SM, Aramideh M, et al. The incidence of cerebral venous thrombosis: a cross-sectional study. Stroke 2012;43(12):3375–7.

7. Devasagayam S, Wyatt B, Leyden J, et al. Cerebral Venous Sinus Thrombosis Incidence Is Higher Than Previously Thought. Stroke 2016;47(9):2180–2.

8. Zhou LW, Yu AYX, Ngo L, et al. Incidence of Cerebral Venous Thrombosis: A Population-Based Study, Systematic Review, and Meta-Analysis. Stroke 2023;54(1):169–77.

9. Capecchi M, Abbattista M, Martinelli I. Cerebral venous sinus thrombosis. J Thromb Haemostasis 2018;16(10):1918–31.

10. Siva A, Altintas A, Saip S. Behcet's syndrome and the nervous system. Curr Opin Neurol 2004;17(3):347–57.

11. Duman T, Demirci S, Uluduz D, et al. Cerebral Venous Sinus Thrombosis as a Rare Complication of Systemic Lupus Erythematosus: Subgroup Analysis of the VENOST Study. J Stroke Cerebrovasc Dis 2019;28(12):104372.

12. Bensalah M, Squizzato A, Ould Kablia S, et al. Cerebral vein and sinus thrombosis and hyperthyrodism: a case report and a systematic review of the literature. Thromb Res 2011;128(1):98–100.

13. Ulivi L, Squitieri M, Cohen H, et al. Cerebral venous thrombosis: a practical guide. Pract Neurol 2020;20(5):356–67.

14. Levi M, van der Poll T, Schultz M. New insights into pathways that determine the link between infection and thrombosis. Neth J Med 2012;70(3):114–20.

15. Schaller B, Graf R. Cerebral venous infarction: the pathophysiological concept. Cerebrovasc Dis 2004;18(3):179–88.

16. Renowden S. Cerebral venous sinus thrombosis. Eur Radiol 2004;14(2):215–26.

17. Wasay M, Kojan S, Dai AI, et al. Headache in Cerebral Venous Thrombosis: incidence, pattern and location in 200 consecutive patients. J Headache Pain 2010;11(2):137–9.

18. de Bruijn SF, Stam J, Kappelle LJ. Thunderclap headache as first symptom of cerebral venous sinus thrombosis. CVST Study Group. Lancet 1996;348(9042):1623–5.

19. Idiculla PS, Gurala D, Palanisamy M, et al. Cerebral Venous Thrombosis: A Comprehensive Review. Eur Neurol 2020;83(4):369–79.

20. Goyal M, Fladt J, Coutinho JM, et al. Endovascular treatment for cerebral venous thrombosis: current status, challenges, and opportunities. J Neurointerventional Surg 2022;14(8):788–93.

21. Tsai LK, Jeng JS, Liu HM, et al. Intracranial dural arteriovenous fistulas with or without cerebral sinus thrombosis: analysis of 69 patients. J Neurol Neurosurg Psychiatr 2004;75(11):1639–41.

22. Ferro JM, Aguiar de Sousa D. Cerebral Venous Thrombosis: an Update. Curr Neurol Neurosci Rep 2019;19(10):74.

23. Coutinho JM, van den Berg R, Zuurbier SM, et al. Small juxtacortical hemorrhages in cerebral venous thrombosis. Ann Neurol 2014;75(6):908–16.

24. Al-Sulaiman A. Clinical Aspects, Diagnosis and Management of Cerebral Vein and Dural Sinus Thrombosis: A Literature Review. Saudi J Med Med Sci 2019;7(3):137–45.

25. Ghoneim A, Straiton J, Pollard C, et al. Imaging of cerebral venous thrombosis. Clin Radiol 2020;75(4):254–64.

26. Virapongse C, Cazenave C, Quisling R, et al. The empty delta sign: frequency and significance in 76 cases of dural sinus thrombosis. Radiology 1987;162(3):779–85.

27. Chik Y, Gottesman RF, Zeiler SR, et al. Differentiation of transverse sinus thrombosis from congenitally atretic cerebral transverse sinus with CT. Stroke 2012;43(7):1968–70.

28. Ferro JM, Bousser MG, Canhão P, et al. European Stroke Organization guideline for the diagnosis and treatment of cerebral venous thrombosis - endorsed by the European Academy of Neurology. Eur J Neurol 2017;24(10):1203–13.

29. Aguiar de Sousa D, Lucas Neto L, Canhão P, et al. Recanalization in Cerebral Venous Thrombosis. Stroke 2018;49(8):1828–35.

30. Einhäupl KM, Villringer A, Meister W, et al. Heparin treatment in sinus venous thrombosis. Lancet 1991;338(8767):597–600.

31. de Bruijn SF, Stam J. Randomized, placebo-controlled trial of anticoagulant treatment with low-molecular-weight heparin for cerebral sinus thrombosis. Stroke 1999;30(3):484–8.

32. Robertson L, Jones LE. Fixed dose subcutaneous low molecular weight heparins versus adjusted dose unfractionated heparin for the initial treatment of venous thromboembolism. Cochrane Database Syst Rev 2017;2(2):Cd001100.

33. Ferro JM, Coutinho JM, Dentali F, et al. Safety and Efficacy of Dabigatran Etexilate vs Dose-Adjusted Warfarin in Patients With Cerebral Venous Thrombosis: A Randomized Clinical Trial. JAMA Neurol 2019;76(12):1457–65.

34. Lee GKH, Chen VH, Tan CH, et al. Comparing the efficacy and safety of direct oral anticoagulants with vitamin K antagonist in cerebral venous thrombosis. J Thromb Thrombolysis 2020;50(3):724–31.

35. Ferro JM, Canhão P, Stam J, et al. Prognosis of cerebral vein and dural sinus thrombosis: results of the International Study on Cerebral Vein and Dural Sinus Thrombosis (ISCVT). Stroke 2004;35(3):664–70.

36. Styczen H, Tsogkas I, Liman J, et al. Endovascular Mechanical Thrombectomy for Cerebral Venous Sinus Thrombosis: A Single-Center Experience. World Neurosurgery 2019;127:e1097–103.

37. Ilyas A, Chen CJ, Raper DM, et al. Endovascular mechanical thrombectomy for cerebral venous sinus thrombosis: a systematic review. J Neurointerv Surg 2017;9(11):1086–92.

38. Coutinho JM, Zuurbier SM, Bousser M-G, et al. Effect of Endovascular Treatment With Medical Management vs Standard Care on Severe Cerebral Venous Thrombosis: The TO-ACT Randomized Clinical Trial. JAMA Neurol 2020;77(8):966–73.

39. Siddiqui FM, Banerjee C, Zuurbier SM, et al. Mechanical thrombectomy versus intrasinus thrombolysis for cerebral venous sinus thrombosis: a non-randomized comparison. Interv Neuroradiol 2014;20(3):336–44.

40. Lee SK, Mokin M, Hetts SW, et al. Current endovascular strategies for cerebral venous thrombosis: report of the SNIS Standards and Guidelines Committee. J Neurointerv Surg 2018;10(8):803–10.

41. Mokin M, Lopes DK, Binning MJ, et al. Endovascular treatment of cerebral venous thrombosis: Contemporary multicenter experience. Interv Neuroradiol 2015;21(4):520–6.

42. Canhão P, Falcão F, Ferro JM. Thrombolytics for cerebral sinus thrombosis: a systematic review. Cerebrovasc Dis 2003;15(3):159–66.

43. Persson L, Lilja A. Extensive dural sinus thrombosis treated by surgical removal and local streptokinase infusion. Neurosurgery 1990;26(1):117–21.

44. Canhão P, Ferro JM, Lindgren AG, et al. Causes and predictors of death in cerebral venous thrombosis. Stroke 2005;36(8):1720–5.

45. Ferro JM, Crassard I, Coutinho JM, et al. Decompressive surgery in cerebrovenous thrombosis: a multicenter registry and a systematic review of individual patient data. Stroke 2011;42(10):2825–31.

46. Aaron S, Alexander M, Moorthy RK, et al. Decompressive craniectomy in cerebral venous thrombosis: a single centre experience. J Neurol Neurosurg Psychiatry 2013;84(9):995–1000.

47. Keller E, Pangalu A, Fandino J, et al. Decompressive craniectomy in severe cerebral venous and dural sinus thrombosis. Acta Neurochir Suppl 2005;94: 177–83.

48. Uluduz D, Midi I, Duman T, et al. Epileptic seizures in cerebral venous sinus thrombosis: Subgroup analysis of VENOST study. Seizure : the journal of the British Epilepsy Association 2020;78:113–7.

49. Ameri A, Bousser MG. Cerebral venous thrombosis. Neurol Clin 1992;10(1):87–111.

50. Murdock J, Tzu JH, Schatz NJ, et al. Optic nerve sheath fenestration for the treatment of papilledema secondary to cerebral venous thrombosis. J Neuro Ophthalmol 2014;34(1):67–9.

51. Standridge SM, O'Brien SH. Idiopathic intracranial hypertension in a pediatric population: a retrospective analysis of the initial imaging evaluation. J Child Neurol 2008;23(11):1308–11.

52. Laurichesse Delmas H, Winer N, Gallot D, et al. Prenatal diagnosis of thrombosis of the dural sinuses: report of six cases, review of the literature and suggested management. Ultrasound Obstet Gynecol 2008;32(2):188–98.

53. Dlamini N, Billinghurst L, Kirkham FJ. Cerebral venous sinus (sinovenous) thrombosis in children. Neurosurg Clin N Am 2010;21(3):511–27.

54. Dakay K, Cooper J, Bloomfield J, et al. Cerebral Venous Sinus Thrombosis in COVID-19 Infection: A Case Series and Review of The Literature. J Stroke Cerebrovasc Dis 2021;30(1):105434.

55. Medicherla CB, Pauley RA, de Havenon A, et al. Cerebral Venous Sinus Thrombosis in the COVID-19 Pandemic. J Neuro Ophthalmol 2020;40(4):457–62.

56. McCullough-Hicks ME, Halterman DJ, Anderson D, et al. High Incidence and Unique Features of Cerebral Venous Sinus Thrombosis in Hospitalized Patients With COVID-19 Infection. Stroke 2022;53(9): e407–10.

57. Cines DB, Bussel JB. SARS-CoV-2 Vaccine-Induced Immune Thrombotic Thrombocytopenia. N Engl J Med 2021;384(23):2254–6.

58. Kowarz E, Krutzke L, Kulp M, et al. Vaccine-induced COVID-19 mimicry syndrome. Elife 2022;11. https://doi.org/10.7554/eLife.74974.

59. Palaiodimou L, Stefanou MI, de Sousa DA, et al. Cerebral venous sinus thrombosis in the setting of COVID-19 vaccination: a systematic review and meta-analysis. J Neurol 2022;269(7):3413–9.

60. Jaiswal V, Nepal G, Dijamco P, et al. Cerebral Venous Sinus Thrombosis Following COVID-19 Vaccination: A Systematic Review. J Prim Care Community Health 2022;13. 21501319221074450.

61. Sriwastava S, Sharma K, Khalid SH, et al. COVID-19 Vaccination and Neurological Manifestations: A Review of Case Reports and Case Series. Brain Sci 2022;12(3). https://doi.org/10.3390/brainsci12030407.

62. Rizk JG, Gupta A, Sardar P, et al. Clinical Characteristics and Pharmacological Management of COVID-19 Vaccine-Induced Immune Thrombotic Thrombocytopenia With Cerebral Venous Sinus Thrombosis: A Review. JAMA Cardiol 2021;6(12):1451–60.

Developmental Venous Anomalies

Li Ma, MD, PhD[a], Samer S. Hoz, MD[a], Jonathan A. Grossberg, MD[b], Michael J. Lang, MD[a], Bradley A. Gross, MD[a],*

KEYWORDS

- Developmental venous anomaly • Venous angioma • Vascular malformation • Venous malformation

KEY POINTS

- Developmental venous anomalies (DVAs) are generally observed clinically as their interruption can disrupt drainage of normal brain parenchyma and result in edema, venous infarction, and hemorrhage.
- Interval imaging may be considered in younger patients to evaluate the potential development of cerebral cavernous malformations in association with DVAs.
- Preservation of DVAs is strongly recommended in the surgical or radiosurgical treatment of associated lesions.

INTRODUCTION

Developmental venous anomalies (DVAs) are relatively common vascular malformations comprised of thickened veins arranged in a radial pattern draining into a common distal vein.[1] The radial array of veins is often described as a "caput medusa." The term "DVA" is synonymous with "venous angioma," "venous anomaly," and "venous malformation." As they drain normal parenchyma, they are not in themselves deemed treatment targets; however, they have been implicated in the formation of cerebral cavernous malformations (CCMs) and capillary telangiectasias and are accordingly often found in association with them.[2,3]

Hemorrhage in association with DVAs, potentially a result of thrombosis, has been reported at annual rates ranging from 0.2% to 0.3%[1,4]; however, even in rare cases of hemorrhage, an associated occult CCM should be evaluated as a potential cause and may even "inflate" these already-low, historical perceived rates of DVA-associated hemorrhage. Since treatment of DVAs would effectively result in thrombosis of the malformation, resultant edema, and potential hemorrhage in the parenchyma that the lesion drains, DVAs should not be viewed as treatment targets.[4,5]

ASSESSMENT/EVALUATION

DVAs are nearly ubiquitously discovered incidentally on contrast-enhanced computed tomography (CT) or MRI. Rarely, a clinical assessment may unveil an association with symptomatology.

Symptomatic Developmental Venous Anomaly Associated with Flow Restriction and/or Mass Effect

Symptomatic DVAs associated with flow restriction and mass effect are relatively rare. In a population-based study, it was found that 98% of DVAs were detected incidentally, with only 2% being potentially symptomatic.[6] This 2% rate is likely further inflated by associated CCM hemorrhage or incidental findings.

DVAs may represent a more delicate venous drainage system susceptible to alterations because

a Department of Neurological Surgery, University of Pittsburgh Medical Center, University of Pittsburgh School of Medicine, Pittsburgh, PA 15213, USA; b Department of Neurological Surgery, Emory University, Atlanta, GA 30322, USA
* Corresponding author. Department of Neurological Surgery, University of Pittsburgh Medical Center, University of Pittsburgh School of Medicine, 200 Lothrop Street, Suite B-400, Pittsburgh, PA 15213.
E-mail address: grossb2@upmc.edu

Neurosurg Clin N Am 35 (2024) 355–361
https://doi.org/10.1016/j.nec.2024.02.007
1042-3680/24/© 2024 Elsevier Inc. All rights reserved.

anatomically, they are variations of normal venous drainage. Most hemorrhages that are associated with DVAs are related to concomitant CCMs rather than the DVA themselves. Very rarely, they may also be associated with a micro-arteriovenous (AV) shunt, which can be diagnosed through angiography and potentially treated through endovascular interventions.[7] Another rare cause of hemorrhage is mechanical obstruction to venous drainage from a DVA that can occur due to anatomic outflow obstructions, such as stenosis or thrombosis of the DVA. These obstructions may present with either intraparenchymal or subarachnoid hemorrhage. More often, these lesions present with venous congestion accompanied by edema. Clinical symptoms may include neurologic deficits, headaches, seizures, and alteration in consciousness or mental status.[7] Thrombosis of the venous drainage is the most common form of mechanical obstruction, followed by either stenosis at some point along the DVAs drainage or complete thrombosis of the DVA in the presence of systemic procoagulation factors, such as in women during the puerperium.[7]

The main draining vein of a DVA can rarely exert mechanical effects on adjacent structures, leading to obstructive or compressive mass effect. In the posterior fossa, collector veins near the root entry zone of cranial nerves may give rise to neurovascular compression such as trigeminal neuralgia. Procedures for neurovascular decompression require special attention because the venous wall of the DVA collector vein is more fragile than that of an arterial vessel and must be preserved. On rare occasions, the DVA collector vein can obstruct cerebrospinal fluid (CSF) flow at the cerebral aqueduct.[8] Depending on the degree of obstruction and the resulting hydrocephalus, either CSF shunting or endoscopic ventriculostomy CSF diversion procedures may be necessary as treatment options.[9]

Association with Cerebral Cavernous Malformations

DVAs exhibit an association with the development of sporadic CCM. The prevalence of associated CCMs in patients with DVAs appears to increase with age, with a prevalence of 0.8% in individuals aged 0 to 10 years, 1.6% in those aged 11 to 20 years, 6.3% to 9.5% in those aged 21 to 70 years, and 11.6% in individuals aged older than 70 years.[10] Sporadic CCMs typically cluster around the draining territory of the collecting vein in patients with DVAs, a pattern distinct from familial CCM cases.[11] Notably, high-sensitivity brain imaging techniques, such as 7 Tesla (7T) MRI, have consistently revealed abnormal venous

drainage in association with sporadic CCMs,[12] thus supporting a pathogenic link between DVAs and CCMs.

Recent genetic investigations have identified somatic activating PIK3CA mutations in cutaneous and mucosal venous malformations,[13] and similar mutations have now been confirmed in DVAs within the brain.[14] Contemporary genetic insights propose that DVAs may act as genetic primers for sporadic CCMs, following a "two hit" theory.[14] In this model, during brain development, a localized genetic mutation in the PIK3CA gene of a vascular cell gives rise to the DVA. Subsequently, a second mutation in 1 of 4 genes—MAP3K3, CCM1, CCM2, or CCM3—within the DVA area leads to the development of the CCM.

Existing studies have produced conflicting results regarding the impact of an associated DVA on the risk of bleeding from the CCM. Some early cohort studies suggested a higher risk of bleeding when a CCM was associated with a DVA.[15,16] However, a recent study demonstrated an equivalent 5 year risk of hemorrhage in patients with CCMs with DVAs versus without (radiographically apparent) DVAs.[17] Furthermore, patients with identifiable DVAs (ie, those seen on standard 1.5 or 3T contrast-enhanced MRI) may represent one end of the spectrum, but sporadic CCMs without radiographically apparent DVA may still exhibit local venous drainage abnormalities.[18] A meta-analysis did not demonstrate DVAs to be a significant risk factor for CCM hemorrhage.[19] Findings from coronavirus disease 2019 (COVID-19) registries suggest that the presence of a DVA may render sporadic CCMs more susceptible to hemorrhage during COVID-19 infection, potentially a result of hypercoagulability-mediated DVA thrombosis.[20]

IMAGING

DVAs are the most common vascular malformation detected on intracranial cross-sectional imaging, with a prevalence of 5% to 10% in contemporary series.[21–23] Most commonly, DVAs are diagnosed incidentally during contrast-enhanced MRI investigations. The prevalence of DVAs on contrast-enhanced MRI appears to rise with age, ranging from 1.5% in neonates and infants to 7.1% in toddlers and preschool-age individuals, and further increasing to 9.6% in school-age and adult populations.[24]

In comparison to contrast-enhanced MRI, susceptibility-weighted imaging (SWI) has improved sensitivity for DVA detection, ranging from 86% to 96%[25] and has demonstrated superior sensitivity when compared to conventional T2* sequences for identifying vascular structures.[26] Often, a maximum intensity projection (mIP) is generated from the SWI scan over 4 adjacent images, creating an effective 8 mm thick section.[27] These mIP images present a great tool for visualizing vessel connectivity and the special relationships of other structures within the brain vasculature. Consequently, invasive imaging techniques such as conventional digital subtraction angiography are generally unindicated. Furthermore, it is worth noting that 7T MRI offers enhanced sensitivity in detecting smaller sized DVAs that might otherwise not be visible on 3T MRI.[28]

Association with Cerebral Cavernous Malformation

High-resolution imaging (such as 7T MRI) has consistently revealed the presence of a DVA in association with sporadic CCMs.[12] Three distinct morphologic phenotypes of DVAs associated with CCMs have been described using 7T MRI (**Fig. 1A–D**). In only 30% of cases, the observed venous structures conform to the typical appearance of a "caput medusa," referred to as variant I. Additionally, 2 novel recurring anatomic patterns

of DVAs have been identified: variant II encompasses lesions with a single transcerebral or a subpial draining vein, primarily draining the CCM (18%), while variant III consists of multiple transcerebral veins originating from the lesion, forming a reticular structure and draining not only the CCM but also the surrounding brain tissue (52%).[12]

Associated Parenchymal Abnormalities

The brain parenchyma within the venous drainage territory of a DVA can exhibit white matter hyperintensities (WMH).[29] WMH in proximity to a DVA have an incidence of 7.8% and are more commonly observed in a periventricular location relative to the DVA.[30] Metabolic abnormalities can also manifest within the venous drainage territory of a DVA.[31,32] Hypometabolism has been documented in regions corresponding to neurologic symptoms, for example, hypometabolism was observed in the visual tracts in patients with visual symptoms and a corresponding DVA.[33] It is noteworthy that structural abnormalities (eg, WMH) were not evident in patients with abnormalities on functional images,[31,32]

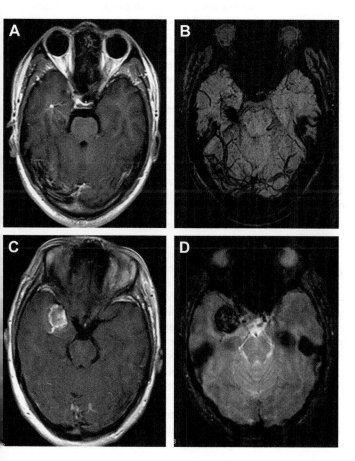

Fig. 1. The variant of the DVA associated with CCM on contrast-enhanced MR and nonenhanced SWI. Demonstrative, postcontrast T1-weighted (*A, C*) and minimum intensity projection images (*B, D*) from 2 patients representing variant type I (*A* and *B*; typical caput medusae) and variant type II (*C* and *D*; singular transcerebral vein) DVAs in the temporal lobe.

underscoring the notion that DVAs have a less robust venous drainage pathway. On rare occasions, DVAs may be observed in regions of cortical developmental malformations, such as polymicrogyria, pachygyria, and focal cortical dysplasia (FCD).[29] Whether the coexistence of these 2 entities is either incidental or due to a shared common insult remains uncertain. Nevertheless, it is important to identify the presence of a DVA in the areas affected by cortical dysplasia, as its inadvertent resection during neurosurgical procedures for an FCD may result in catastrophic venous infarction due to its vulnerability to hemodynamic changes.

MANAGEMENT AND IMPACT ON THE TREATMENT OF ASSOCIATED LESIONS

In general, DVAs are not considered primary targets for therapeutic intervention.[34] Spontaneous hemorrhages attributed to DVAs are infrequent and typically ascribed to underlying factors such as CCMs, venous outflow obstruction, or flow-related shunts, unless proven otherwise. A series of stereotactic radiosurgery (SRS) for DVAs has yielded low obliteration rates and high complication rates.[5] This underscores that SRS is not a suitable treatment option for these anomalies. Microsurgical removal of a DVA, even during the resection of a CCM, is generally not recommended due to the risk of edema, hemorrhage, or infarction. Although some DVAs may be resected without sequelae, there are currently no clinical or radiographic methods to predict whether the resection of a specific DVA will be well tolerated. This point is especially true with brainstem CCMs, where resection of the DVA can lead to a catastrophic neurologic deficit. It is critical to employ vascular imaging and recognize the presence of a DVA, as it can sometimes be either concealed or distorted by the hematoma. When contemplating surgical evacuation of a cerebral hematoma, effort should be made to preserve the DVA.[35]

Management of Symptomatic Developmental Venous Anomalies

There is currently no compelling evidence to suggest that DVAs are more predisposed to thrombosis than normal cerebral veins. Consequently, conservative management without anticoagulation or antiplatelet therapy remains the prevailing approach. Overall, favorable outcomes have been observed in 82.8% of patients with presumed, symptomatic DVA.

In very rare cases of definitive thrombosis in the confirmed absence of an associated vascular malformation, systemic heparinization has been administered, akin to treatment strategies for sinus or cerebral venous thrombosis.[36,37] However, standard precautions for initiating anticoagulation must be observed and should be avoided when there is a coexisting CCM, given the potential risk of bleeding. In rare instances, decompressive craniectomy may be necessary for refractory and malignant regional edema, or ventricular shunt placement for ensuing hydrocephalus may be indicated.

Developmental Venous Anomalies in the Management of Associated Cerebral Cavernous Malformation

Current data suggest that sporadic CCMs with radiographically apparent, associated DVAs do not harbor an increased risk of hemorrhage or resultant size of hemorrhage should bleeding occur. Therefore, the presence of a DVA on standard MRI (1.5 or 3T contrast-enhanced) should not serve as an indication for proceeding with surgical resection of a CCM. While some earlier reports suggested the surgical removal of the associated DVA based on concerns that DVAs may be the primary pathologic lesion leading to recurrent CCMs,[38–41] a consensus among experienced surgeons noted that DVAs must be preserved during surgery.[34,42–45] This consensus is rooted in an understanding that DVAs often represent the normal venous drainage for the region in which they reside, and their obliteration may result in venous congestion or infarction. Given that hemorrhage from CCMs is rarely life threatening, the severe consequences of venous infarction outweigh the risk of CCM recurrence.[46]

Although DVAs of varying degrees may be identified in association with the majority of CCMs on high-resolution MRI, intraoperative identification is estimated to occur in at least half of patients. DVAs exhibit no specific relation to lesion depth and can traverse various directions, either deep or superficial to the lesion. Furthermore, an association has been noted between DVA preservation and neurologic outcomes. Consequently, the presence of a DVA has been incorporated into the surgical outcome grading system of brainstem CCMs.[47] Preservation of DVAs is considered standard practice since they form part of normal venous circulation, and their compromise can cause either venous ischemia or infarction. Radiographically apparent, associated DVAs are speculated to increase the overall complexity of CCM resections, introducing challenges potentially in the surgical corridor, intraoperative bleeding, or even generating satellite lesions in the brainstem.

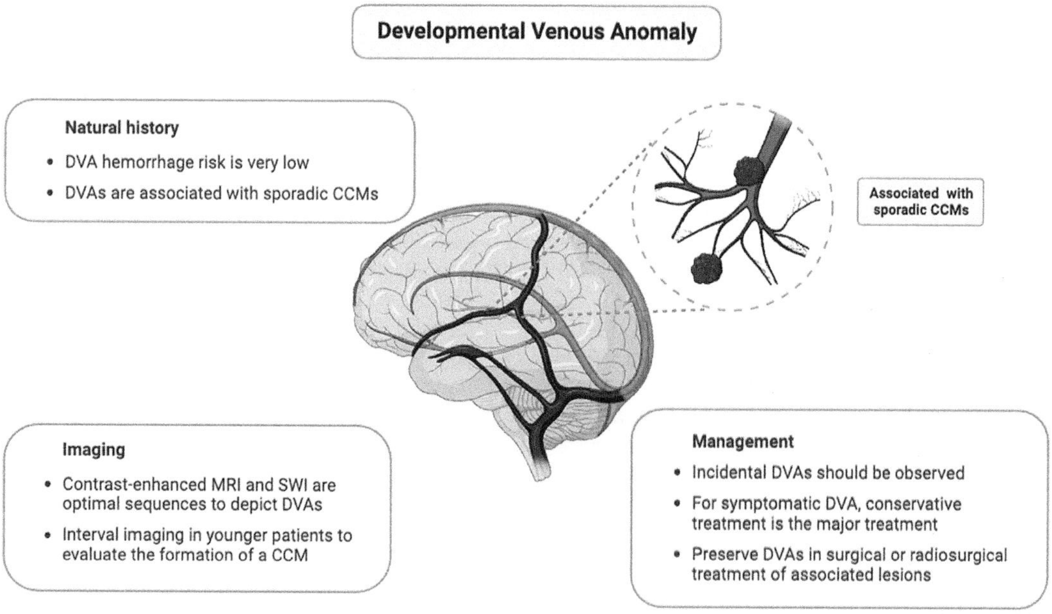

Fig. 2. Summary of clinical care points for DVA.

Although SRS for CCMs is itself controversial, the presence of a DVA has been identified as a risk factor for new hemorrhages after SRS, associated with an approximately 1.6 fold decrease in the presumed efficacy of SRS for CCMs.[48] If SRS is performed, it is recommended to exclude the area of the DVA from the isodose line by using conformal treatment methods whenever possible.[49] However, omitting the area of the DVA during radiation treatment may lead to reduced SRS efficacy in cases involving CCMs associated with DVAs.

SUMMARY

DVAs are the most common vascular malformation detected on noninvasive, enhanced intracranial cross-sectional imaging. Although typically benign, DVAs can rarely manifest symptomatically, including either hemorrhage or infarction. However, it is crucial to recognize that spontaneous hemorrhages attributed to DVAs are rare and should be ascribed to underlying factors such as associated CCMs, flow-related shunts, or venous outflow obstruction. Imaging modalities such as contrast-enhanced MRI, SWI, and high-field MRI provide great tools for visualizing vessel connectivity and the special relationships of other structures. DVAs are not typically targeted for therapeutic intervention. The preservation of DVAs is a well-established practice in the surgical or radiosurgical treatment of associated lesions (**Fig. 2**).

CLINICS CARE POINTS

- The risk of hemorrhage associated with DVAs is generally very low; however, it can be linked to sporadic CCMs and collecting vein thrombosis.
- Contrast-enhanced MRI and SWI serve as great tools for visualizing DVAs and assessing the presence of associated CCMs.
- Incidental identification of DVAs does not warrant therapeutic intervention.
- In cases of symptomatic DVAs, conservative management is the primary approach.
- Preservation of DVAs is strongly recommended in the surgical or radiosurgical treatment of associated lesions.

DISCLOSURE

This study did not receive any funding or financial support. Dr B.A. Gross is a consultant for Medtronic, Stryker, and MicroVention.

REFERENCES

1. Garner TB, Del Curling O Jr, Kelly DL Jr, et al. The natural history of intracranial venous angiomas. J Neurosurg 1991;75(5):715–22.
2. Rigamonti D, Johnson PC, Spetzler RF, et al. Cavernous malformations and capillary telangiectasia:

a spectrum within a single pathological entity. Neurosurgery 1991;28(1):60–4.

3. Abla A, Wait SD, Uschold T, et al. Developmental venous anomaly, cavernous malformation, and capillary telangiectasia: spectrum of a single disease. Acta Neurochir (Wien) 2008;150(5):487–9. discussion 489.

4. McLaughlin MR, Kondziolka D, Flickinger JC, et al. The prospective natural history of cerebral venous malformations. Neurosurgery 1998;43(2):195–200. discussion 200-201.

5. Lindquist C, Guo WY, Karlsson B, et al. Radiosurgery for venous angiomas. J Neurosurg 1993; 78(4):531–6.

6. Hon JM, Bhattacharya JJ, Counsell CE, et al. The presentation and clinical course of intracranial developmental venous anomalies in adults: a systematic review and prospective, population-based study. Stroke 2009;40(6):1980–5.

7. Pereira VM, Geibprasert S, Krings T, et al. Pathomechanisms of symptomatic developmental venous anomalies. Stroke 2008;39(12):3201–15.

8. Blackmore CC, Mamourian AC. Aqueduct compression from venous angioma: MR findings. AJNR Am J Neuroradiol 1996;17(3):458–60.

9. Xian Z, Fung SH, Nakawah MO. Obstructive hydrocephalus due to aqueductal stenosis from developmental venous anomaly draining bilateral medial thalami: a case report. Radiol Case Rep 2020; 15(6):730–2.

10. Brinjikji W, El-Masri AE, Wald JT, et al. Prevalence of cerebral cavernous malformations associated with developmental venous anomalies increases with age. Childs Nerv Syst 2017;33(9):1539–43.

11. Dammann P, Wrede K, Zhu Y, et al. Correlation of the venous angioarchitecture of multiple cerebral cavernous malformations with familial or sporadic disease: a susceptibility-weighted imaging study with 7-Tesla MRI. J Neurosurg 2017;126(2):570–7.

12. Dammann P, Wrede KH, Maderwald S, et al. The venous angioarchitecture of sporadic cerebral cavernous malformations: a susceptibility weighted imaging study at 7 T MRI. J Neurol Neurosurg Psychiatry 2013;84(2):194–200.

13. Limaye N, Kangas J, Mendola A, et al. Somatic Activating PIK3CA Mutations Cause Venous Malformation. Am J Hum Genet 2015;97(6):914–21.

14. Snellings DA, Girard R, Lightle R, et al. Developmental venous anomalies are a genetic primer for cerebral cavernous malformations. Nat Cardiovasc Res 2022;1:246–52.

15. Kashefiolasl S, Bruder M, Brawanski N, et al. A benchmark approach to hemorrhage risk management of cavernous malformations. Neurology 2018;90(10):e856–63.

16. Tian KB, Zheng JJ, Ma JP, et al. Clinical course of untreated thalamic cavernous malformations: hemorrhage

risk and neurological outcomes. J Neurosurg 2017; 127(3):480–91.

17. Gross BA, Du R. Hemorrhage from cerebral cavernous malformations: a systematic pooled analysis. J Neurosurg 2017;126(4):1079–87.

18. Shkoukani A, Srinath A, Stadnik A, et al. COVID-19 in a Hemorrhagic Neurovascular Disease, Cerebral Cavernous Malformation. J Stroke Cerebrovasc Dis 2021;30(11):106101.

19. Chen B, Herten A, Saban D, et al. Hemorrhage from cerebral cavernous malformations: The role of associated developmental venous anomalies. Neurology 2020;95(1):e89–96.

20. Rabinstein AA, Flemming KD. Cavernous malformations with DVA: Hold those knives. Neurology 2020; 95(1):13–4.

21. Jones BV, Linscott L, Koberlein G, et al. Increased Prevalence of Developmental Venous Anomalies in Children with Intracranial Neoplasms. AJNR Am J Neuroradiol 2015;36(9):1782–5.

22. Linscott LL, Leach JL, Jones BV, et al. Developmental venous anomalies of the brain in children – imaging spectrum and update. Pediatr Radiol 2016;46(3):394–406. quiz 391-393.

23. Gokce E, Acu B, Beyhan M, et al. Magnetic resonance imaging findings of developmental venous anomalies. Clin Neuroradiol 2014;24(2):135–43.

24. Brinjikji W, El-Rida El-Masri A, Wald JT, et al. Prevalence of Developmental Venous Anomalies Increases With Age. Stroke 2017;48(7):1997–9.

25. Young A, Poretti A, Bosemani T, et al. Sensitivity of susceptibility-weighted imaging in detecting developmental venous anomalies and associated cavernomas and microhemorrhages in children. Neuroradiology 2017;59(8):797–802.

26. Tsui YK, Tsai FY, Hasso AN, et al. Susceptibility-weighted imaging for differential diagnosis of cerebral vascular pathology: a pictorial review. J Neurol Sci 2009;287(1–2):7–16.

27. Haacke EM, Mittal S, Wu Z, et al. Susceptibility-weighted imaging: technical aspects and clinical applications, part 1. AJNR Am J Neuroradiol 2009; 30(1):19–30.

28. Frischer JM, God S, Gruber A, et al. Susceptibility-weighted imaging at 7 T: Improved diagnosis of cerebral cavernous malformations and associated developmental venous anomalies. Neuroimage Clin 2012;1(1):116–20.

29. Hsu CC, Krings T. Symptomatic Developmental Venous Anomaly: State-of-the-Art Review on Genetics, Pathophysiology, and Imaging Approach to Diagnosis. AJNR Am J Neuroradiol 2023;44(5):498–504.

30. Santucci GM, Leach JL, Ying J, et al. Brain parenchymal signal abnormalities associated with developmental venous anomalies: detailed MR imaging assessment. AJNR Am J Neuroradiol 2008;29(7): 1317–23.

31. Larvie M, Timerman D, Thum JA. Brain metabolic abnormalities associated with developmental venous anomalies. AJNR Am J Neuroradiol 2015; 36(3):475–80.

32. Lazor JW, Schmitt JE, Loevner LA, et al. Metabolic Changes of Brain Developmental Venous Anomalies on (18)F-FDG-PET. Acad Radiol 2019;26(4):443–9.

33. Imai M, Tanaka M, Ishibashi K, et al. Glucose Hypometabolism in Developmental Venous Anomaly Without Apparent Parenchymal Damage. Clin Nucl Med 2017;42(5):361–3.

34. Naff NJ, Wemmer J, Hoenig-Rigamonti K, et al. A longitudinal study of patients with venous malformations: documentation of a negligible hemorrhage risk and benign natural history. Neurology 1998; 50(6):1709–14.

35. Nagatani K, Osada H, Takeuchi S, et al. Surgical resection of developmental venous anomaly causing massive intracerebral haemorrhage: a case report. Br J Neurosurg 2014;28(1):116–8.

36. Agazzi S, Regli L, Uske A, et al. Developmental venous anomaly with an arteriovenous shunt and a thrombotic complication. Case report. J Neurosurg 2001;94(3):533–7.

37. Lovrencic-Huzjan A, Rumboldt Z, Marotti M, et al. Subarachnoid haemorrhage headache from a developmental venous anomaly. Cephalalgia 2004; 24(9):763–6.

38. Labauge P, Brunereau L, Levy C, et al. The natural history of familial cerebral cavernomas: a retrospective MRI study of 40 patients. Neuroradiology 2000; 42(5):327–32.

39. Biller J, Toffol GJ, Shea JF, et al. Cerebellar venous angiomas. A continuing controversy. Arch Neurol 1985;42(4):367–70.

40. Denier C, Labauge P, Bergametti F, et al. Genotype-phenotype correlations in cerebral cavernous malformations patients. Ann Neurol 2006;60(5):550–6.

41. Malik GM, Morgan JK, Boulos RS, et al. Venous angiomas: an underestimated cause of intracranial hemorrhage. Surg Neurol 1988;30(5):350–8.

42. Porter RW, Detwiler PW, Spetzler RF, et al. Cavernous malformations of the brainstem: experience with 100 patients. J Neurosurg 1999;90(1):50–8.

43. Zimmerman RS, Spetzler RF, Lee KS, et al. Cavernous malformations of the brain stem. J Neurosurg 1991;75(1):32–9.

44. Rigamonti D, Spetzler RF. The association of venous and cavernous malformations. Report of four cases and discussion of the pathophysiological, diagnostic, and therapeutic implications. Acta Neurochir (Wien) 1988;92(1–4):100–5.

45. Sasaki O, Tanaka R, Koike T, et al. Excision of cavernous angioma with preservation of coexisting venous angioma. Case report. J Neurosurg 1991; 75(3):461–4.

46. Barrow DL, Schuette AJ. Cavernous malformations: a paradigm for progress. Clin Neurosurg 2011;58: 27–41.

47. Garcia RM, Ivan ME, Lawton MT. Brainstem cavernous malformations: surgical results in 104 patients and a proposed grading system to predict neurological outcomes. Neurosurgery 2015;76(3): 265–77. discussion 277-268.

48. Dumot C, Mantziaris G, Dayawansa S, et al. Stereotactic radiosurgery for haemorrhagic cerebral cavernous malformation: a multi-institutional, retrospective study. Stroke Vasc Neurol 2023;svn(2023): 002380.

49. Karaaslan B, Gulsuna B, Erol G, et al. Stereotactic radiosurgery for cerebral cavernous malformation: comparison of hemorrhage rates before and after stereotactic radiosurgery. J Neurosurg 2022; 136(3):655–61.

Vein of Galen Malformations

Alex Devarajan, BS, Daryl Goldman, MD, Tomoyoshi Shigematsu, MD, PhD,
Alejandro Berenstein, MD, Johanna T. Fifi, MD*

KEYWORDS

- Vein of Galen malformation • Embolization • Transvenous • Transarterial
- Arteriovenous malformation • Congenital vascular malformation

KEY POINTS

- Neonatal patients with vein of Galen malformations (VOGMs) are often diagnosed antenatally but require comprehensive workup to assess their cardiac and neurologic prognosis and the need for emergent neonatal embolization to control refractory symptoms.
- Infantile patients with VOGM often present with more neurologic symptoms and require close follow-up with their pediatrician to monitor for any new or worsening symptoms suggestive of a VOGM.
- Staged transarterial embolization (TAE) is the gold standard of endovascular management of the VOGM. Embolizations must be scheduled to balance time for hemodynamic remodeling of the malformation against the development of complicating angiogenesis in the malformation.
- Transvenous embolization may be considered for a final curative embolization after progressive reductions of the shunt from staged TAE. Neurosurgical interventions are limited to adjunctive relief of hydrocephalus.
- Comprehensive genomic and transcriptomic studies have begun to define key molecular markers in patients which may serve as future therapeutic targets.

INTRODUCTION

Vein of Galen malformations (VOGMs) are congenital brain arteriovenous malformations (AVMs) characterized by maldevelopment of the intracranial midline venous system.[1–3] VOGMs represent about 1% of cerebrovascular malformations but comprise approximately 30% of pediatric cerebrovascular malformations.[4] VOGMs develop between weeks 6 and 11 of gestation and are characterized by high-flow fistulas between the choroidal circulation and the median prosencephalic vein of Markowski (MPV), the embryonic precursor to the vein of Galen.[5] No known risk factors exist for the development of VOGM, though a genetic cause has been increasingly suggested.[6,7] The initial clinical manifestations of VOGM are variable: they range from asymptomatic to severe heart failure in the neonate to macrocephaly, seizures, and developmental delays in infants and young children.[3,8] Symptomatic VOGMs, if left untreated, have a mortality rate of 76.7%.[9] Endovascular embolization is the definitive first-line therapy for VOGM management; the historic mortality rate after microsurgical intervention was near 100%, while the mortality in patients who receive endovascular embolization has improved over time to approximately 15.7% of all patients.[2,3,10] Advancements in early diagnosis, imaging, multidisciplinary care across pediatric subspecialties, endovascular embolization technology and techniques, and understanding of the pathophysiology have all contributed to the increased likelihood of patients remaining at neurologic baseline and

Department of Neurosurgery, Icahn School of Medicine at Mount Sinai, New York, NY, USA
* Corresponding author. Department of Neurosurgery, Icahn School of Medicine at Mount Sinai, 1450 Madison Avenue, Floor 1-North, New York, NY 10029.
E-mail address: Johanna.fifi@mountsinai.org
Twitter: @johannatfifi (J.T.F.)

Neurosurg Clin N Am 35 (2024) 363–374
https://doi.org/10.1016/j.nec.2024.02.008
1042-3680/24/© 2024 Elsevier Inc. All rights reserved.

leading relatively normal lives. In this article, we discuss the pathophysiology, embryology, angioarchitecture, diagnostic evaluation, medical management, endovascular management, surgical management, prognosis, and future directions in our understanding of VOGM.

EMBRYOLOGY, PATHOPHYSIOLOGY, AND ANGIOARCHITECTURE

VOGM is an embryonic choroid plexus AVM, distinct from other deep-seated AVMs with venous drainage into a more mature vein of Galen.[3] Early in brain development, arterial supply is derived from the choroid plexuses and several associated choroidal arteries while venous drainage primarily occurs through the MPV.[8] In gestational weeks 8 to 11, the MPV segment proximal to its connection with the internal cerebral veins (ICVs) involutes and regresses as the ICVs assume venous drainage of the choroid plexuses.[11,12] The distal MPV segment gives rise to the vein of Galen, and cortical arteries take over arterial supply. However, in VOGM, after the choroidal circulation abnormally connects with the proximal MPV in utero, the increased venous pressure leads to aneurysmal dilatation and prevents normal involution of the proximal MPV. Therefore, the choroidal arterial circulation derived from the prosencephalon and the MPV persist as a low-resistance high-flow intracranial shunt.

The symptoms and findings seen in VOGM can be attributed to its complex pathophysiology (**Table 1**).[13] In the low-resistance fetal circulation, patients with VOGM exhibit high cardiac output which drives increased venous return with associated superior vena cava (SVC) and right-sided dilation.[14] The increased right-sided flow can pass through the ductus arteriosus to the descending aorta, causing excessive net pulmonary blood flow which can predispose to severe pulmonary hypertension. The low-resistance VOGM is balanced by the low-resistance placental circulation. After birth and in the neonatal period, the VOGM with high-output shunting may collect up to 80% of the cardiac output, causing cardiogenic shock.[15] Massively increased cardiac preload and ductus arteriosus closure lead to elevations in pulmonary vascular pressures with severe respiratory distress and eventual persistent pulmonary hypertension of the newborn (PPHN). Cardiomegaly with reduced biventricular systolic function occurs due to intraventricular septal displacement and increased preload. The patient develops arterial hypotension and venous hypertension, leading to diastolic flow reversal across the aorta. This arterial hypotension drives "steal" from the cerebral circulation, which prevents the

normal postnatal physiologic increase in brain perfusion and leads to bihemispheric brain injuries with intracranial venous congestion.[16] Coronary artery flow is decreased but cardiac metabolic demand continues to increase, leading to myocardial ischemia and high-output heart failure. This leads to multiorgan failure with associated systemic hypotension, hepatomegaly, and renal failure. In lower output shunts or with venous outflow restriction, patients may not develop severe heart failure and may then present as infants or later due to symptoms of persistently increased intracranial venous congestion.[3,17]

Considering their embryology, arterial feeders to the VOGM can be generally categorized as prosencephalic arteries (including anterior choroidal, posterior choroidal, and pericallosal arteries) or transmesencephalic arteries (including thalamoperforating branches) arising from the proximal posterior cerebral arteries and basilar tip.[8] Other feeding vessels including the middle cerebral artery, superior cerebellar artery, and meningeal branches can be seen. Lasjaunias and colleagues classified VOGMs into choroidal VOGM (with a nidus-like arterial feeding network) and mural VOGM (with 1 or 2 direct fistulous arteries) to inform treatment approach and difficulty, but rates of good neurologic outcome are comparable.[3] Venous drainage typically occurs through a persistent falcine sinus in the posterior falx cerebri to normal venous sinuses, as the straight sinus may be hypoplastic or entirely absent. Collateral venous drainage may be present along with a persistent occipital sinus. Deep venous drainage from the ICVs into the VOGM is a high-risk feature present in approximately 33% of patients.[18] Occlusion of these vessels with resultant secondary venous congestion can cause significant iatrogenic morbidity and mortality. Postembolization angiography is crucial to assess for stasis in the ICVs suggestive of occlusion. In a subset of patients, later in infancy and childhood, stenosis of the sigmoid–jugular junction and transverse sinus can occur, leading to retrograde venous drainage and collateral venous outflow often into the cavernous sinus and facial veins.[19]

Single-center series have described the development of marked angiogenesis in approximately 60% of patients (**Fig. 1**A–D).[20] VOGMs recruit dural collaterals similar to other AVMs and arteriovenous fistulas, but additionally exhibit extra-axial angiogenesis forming an extensive plexiform network of collateral vasculature within the subarachnoid spaces and quadrigeminal cisterns, which complicates treatment in select patients.[2,20,21] Several hypotheses have been proposed, including local hypoxia, inflammation, and hemodynamic wall

Table 1
Symptoms by organ system and age

System	Antenatal	Neonatal	Infantile
Systemic	• Hydrops fetalis • Anasarca	• Failure to thrive • Macrocephaly • Full fontanelles • Visible scalp veins	• Macrocephaly • Full fontanelles • Visible scalp veins

Cardiac	• Pericardial effusion
	• Cardiomegaly
		• High-output heart failure
		• Cardiogenic shock
		• Cardiomegaly
		• Cranial bruit
		• Congenital heart defects:[13]
		  ○ Atrial septal defects
		  ○ Aortic coarctation
		  ○ Aortic hypoplasia	

Neurologic		• Seizures • Ischemic brain injury • Communicating hydrocephalus • Upward gaze palsy	• Communicating hydrocephalus • Headaches • Upward gaze palsy • Developmental delay/regression • Focal neurologic deficits

Respiratory	• Pleural effusion	• Pulmonary hypertension
		• Tachypnea
		• Cyanosis
		• Respiratory distress
		  ○ Nasal flaring
		  ○ Chest retractions
		  ○ Poor feeding	

Hepatic		• Hepatomegaly • Liver failure (abnormal LFTs)	
Renal		• Renal failure • Decreased urine output • Anuria	

stress, but no definitive answer has been identified.[22] Current and future studies have highlighted molecular drivers of arterial and venous differentiation in endothelial cells to understand molecular drivers of VOGM and vasculogenesis.

DIAGNOSIS AND EVALUATION

The majority of neonatal VOGMs in developed countries are diagnosed antenatally on third trimester maternal ultrasound.[1] Fetal distress, presenting as cardiac insufficiency or hydrops fetalis on imaging, or acute postnatal cardiopulmonary distress with associated multiorgan dysfunction are often seen in neonatal VOGM.[3] The initial clinical evaluation of neonates involves a complete neurologic examination, head circumference measurements, vascular access with preservation of the umbilical arteries, fontanelle auscultation and ultrasound, chest radiographs, and prompt evaluation of cardiac function by bedside transthoracic echocardiogram.[23] The newborn may exhibit increased work of breathing or respiratory

distress. Chest radiograph will quickly identify cardiomegaly and pulmonary vascular congestion.[23] Echocardiogram will identify comorbid congenital heart disease and rule out cyanotic congenital heart disease or intracardiac causes of heart failure which present similarly to VOGM.[13] Echocardiograms should explicitly assess direction and amount of blood flow through the great vessels with antegrade : retrograde velocity time integral (VTI) ratios and measurement of chamber and vessel diameters (**Box 1**). Neonates in distress should be empirically screened for heart failure with brain natriuretic peptide levels, arterial blood gas (ABG) with lactate, and electrocardiogram.[29] Multiorgan function should be assessed with a comprehensive metabolic panel including liver and renal function testing. Neuroimaging is mandatory as part of the neonatal assessment (**Table 2**). Brain MRI should be obtained to characterize the lesion and assess for cortical damage or melting brain syndrome. Bedside electroencephalography (EEG) may be employed if there is clinical concern for seizure. The Bicetre neonatal

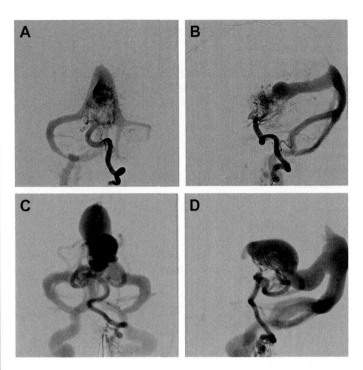

Fig. 1. Subtracted anteroposterior (AP) (*A*) and lateral (*B*) views of the left vertebral artery in a 13 month old patient demonstrate a fine collateral network of vasculature within the third ventricle and choroidal fissure. Subtracted anteroposterior (AP) (*C*) and lateral (*D*) views of the left vertebral artery in another 13 month old patient demonstrate a high-flow VOGM without the presence of any angiogenesis.

evaluation score was proposed by Lasjaunias and colleagues as a basic heuristic for deciding whether to embolize in the neonate by scoring decompensation of cardiac, pulmonary, neurologic, renal, and hepatic function (**Table 3**).[3] This 21 point score and decision-making tool is a guide and not strictly adhered to in the modern era. If embolization is not needed until later in infancy, patients need close follow-up with their pediatrician and cardiology if indicated. Monitoring for signs of cerebral injury with computerized tomography or MRI is necessary to identify indications for earlier treatment, such as development of parenchymal calcifications or hydrocephalus.

Some VOGMs are only diagnosed in the infantile period or later. Careful assessment by parent and pediatrician on routine well-child visits can identify whether a patient is falling off their growth curve for head circumference or deviating from their neurologic baseline, which raises suspicion for underlying intracranial vascular malformations.

MEDICAL MANAGEMENT

The primary goal of neonatal medical management is to stabilize cardiopulmonary and neurologic symptoms until embolization. Bubble continuous positive airway pressure (CPAP) provides efficient mechanical respiratory support to neonates demonstrating an increased work of breathing on room air. If Fio_2 requirements continue to increase

or severe respiratory distress syndrome is demonstrated on chest radiographs or ABG/venous blood gas (VBG), surfactant administration should be considered.[29] If the patient continues to decline, intubation and mechanical ventilation are necessary; if refractory to medical management, emergent neonatal embolization is indicated.

Aggressive management of heart failure with inotropes, diuresis, and vasodilators is indicated in neonates with respiratory failure.[29] Pulmonary hypertension frequently presents as a complicating factor and must be aggressively managed as well.[34] Intravenous milrinone has specific inotropic benefit in neonates with PPHN and can be empirically started if there is concern for severe heart failure.[35] Inhaled nitric oxide has been used for management of PPHN and hypoxemic respiratory failure secondary to AVMs, but its efficacy is debated and it may worsen congestive heart failure in patients with VOGM.[36] Prostaglandin E1 may be considered for further cardiac support and maintenance of a patent ductus arteriosus in patients with heart failure and PPHN.[37] Supportive care should otherwise be initiated to correct metabolic acidosis, hypoglycemia, or anemia that may develop secondary to heart failure while the patient awaits embolization. If indicated, levetiracetam is well tolerated as a first-line therapy for seizure prophylaxis and can be transitioned to the outpatient setting.[38] If alone or with medical management, the neonate is able to breathe on

Echocardiogram Features Suggesting Emergent Embolization

- Moderate-to-severe right ventricular dysfunction
- Moderate-to-severe tricuspid regurgitation[24]
- Diastolic flow reversal across aortic arch (antegrade:retrograde VTI ratio <1)[26]
- Severe pulmonary hypertension (suprasystemic pulmonary artery pressure)[27]
- Elevated SVC:IVC diameter ratio
- Elevated combined cardiac index[25]

Brain MRI Features Suggestive of Emergent Embolization[28]

- Mediolateral diameter of falcine sinus at narrowest point greater than 6.2 mm
- A cross-sectional area of falcine sinus at narrowest point greater than 58 mm^2

Brain MRI Features Suggestive of Nonintervention/Palliative Measures

- Significant parenchymal volume loss (melting brain)
- Extensive intracranial hemorrhage
- Diffuse white matter injury
- Bilateral diffuse parenchymal injury

their own and tolerate feeds, embolization can be deferred to the age of 5 to 8 months when it is technically less challenging and complication risk is lower.

ENDOVASCULAR MANAGEMENT

Endovascular embolization is the cornerstone of VOGM management. The technical goal of embolization is safe and permanent disconnection of fistulas at the inflow of the draining vein. Owing to the complexity of the vascular anatomy and hemodynamics, VOGMs are frequently closed over several embolization sessions.[2] In the neonatal period, with contrast dose and access restraints, targeted MR angiography-guided transarterial procedures to close the largest of the fistulas are the procedure of choice. Umbilical access is favored, while ultrasound-guided percutaneous femoral access is utilized in infants and older children. The umbilical artery catheter can either be exchanged for a 4 French sheath or utilized directly as a sheath and guide catheter for emergent repeat embolizations, but the indwelling catheter must be monitored

for infection. Transfemoral access is the second choice for neonates and may lead to femoral arterial thrombosis which complicates future arterial access. The goal is to close 1 to 3 large fistulas with enough reduction of arterial shunting to stabilize the heart failure. Heart failure is evaluated clinically and with echocardiogram after the procedure. Some patients require multiple embolizations in the neonatal period.

Patients, regardless of prior need for neonatal embolization, undergo angiogram and embolization at about 5 to 8 months of age and often continue in a staged fashion. The goal of these procedures is reduction and closure of the shunt resulting in decreasing size of the aneurysmal vein. These staged sessions are usually planned every 2 to 6 months. Timing of this staging is dependent on the percentage of shunt closed after the current embolization, concern for the development of fine angiogenic networks, and symptom severity. Postembolization angiograms should assess reduction in arteriovenous shunting without venous stagnation or distal emboli. It is important to assess deep venous drainage, as normal venous outflow like the ICVs can be incorporated into the malformation and accidentally occluded iatrogenically (**Fig. 2**).[18] Embolizing aggressively can cause abrupt hemodynamic changes and potential thrombosis within the vein, leading to rupture and catastrophic intracranial hemorrhage. Aiming for staged reduction sessions with breaks allowing for sufficient remodeling of the cerebral vasculature and hypertrophy of remaining pedicles is a safe and effective way to obliterate the VOGM.[2]

Liquid embolic agents (LEAs) such as cyanoacrylates or ethylene-vinyl-alcohol copolymer (EVOH) are the embolic material of choice.[39] Traditionally, flow-directed microcatheters placed distally in the fistula are used for embolization.[40] When injecting embolic material, adjunctive global flow control techniques such as medically induced hypotension or rapid ventricular overdrive pacing can be employed to reduce the risk of venous escape and increase the likelihood of on-target embolization.[41] Detachable tip catheters have been utilized to inject liquid embolic without fear of catheter entrapment in high-flow fistulas. Transarterially placed balloon microcatheters have been recently utilized to provide local flow control for safer embolization while occluding the vessel to prevent retrograde reflux.[42] Coils placed via TAE or transvenous embolization (TVE) into the arterial pedicle at the venous outflow junction can be used with or without adjunctive LEA, but proximal coil placement is detrimental.[43] Somatosensory- and motor-evoked potentials, with occasional

Table 2
Neuroimaging considerations

Ultrasound	• Typical modality to diagnose neonatal VOGM[1] • Maternal: antenatal diagnosis in the third trimester • Cranial: postnatal diagnosis • Superior sagittal sinus: venous congestion[30] • Transfontanellar: cystic encephalomalacia or parenchymal changes[3] • Doppler: median anechoic and dilated venous sac with marked pulsatility posterior to third ventricle[31]

Brain MRI	• Confirm diagnosis after ultrasound
	• Characterize:
	  ○ Aneurysmal dilatation
	  ○ Surrounding parenchymal injury
	  ○ Hydrocephalus
	• Important sequences
	  ○ *T2*: flow voids of aneurysmal dilatation and feeding vessels; brain parenchyma
	  ○ *Diffusion-weighted imaging*: diffusion restriction suggestive of ischemic injury
	  ○ *T2* gradient echo*: blooming suggestive of cortical injury[32]

MR angiography	• Noninvasive characterization of cerebral vasculature and venous outflow • Obtain in conjunction with MRI
Computerized tomography (CT)	• Quick characterization of hydrocephalus • Cross-sectional view of aneurysmal dilatation • Parenchymal calcifications
CT angiography	• Can delineate vasculature • Technically challenging in high-output heart failure: small contrast load and rapid shunting limit use[33] • Not favored for characterization

Digital subtraction angiography (DSA)	• Gold standard for diagnosis
	• Only used if concurrent embolization is planned
	• Characterize:
	  ○ Degree of arteriovenous shunting
	  ○ Size of aneurysmal dilatation
	  ○ Anatomy of arterial feeders
	  ○ Dangerous anastomoses
	  ○ Vascular supply to eloquent brain

provocative testing with sodium methohexital, can be monitored intraprocedurally to protect against intraoperative injury especially when embolizing via perforating arteries. If recent imaging is not available, an MRI should be obtained for procedural planning.

Fine angiogenic networks of collateral vasculature can develop rapidly between embolizations.[2,20] Patients who develop these networks require special consideration, and time between treatment sessions should be decreased to minimize further angiogenesis. Though intervening networks complicate transarterial access, miniature balloon microcatheters provide sufficiently distal access to the malformation.[44] A careful monitoring of the EVOH penetration is necessary to avoid accidental embolization of thalamoperforating arteries or arteries supplying eloquent brain (**Fig. 3**A, B).

TVE may be considered for a final curative embolization after staged TAE when residual feeders are limited to small-caliber thalamoperforating or choroidal arteries.[43] As historically primary transvenous coiling of the venous pouch carries significant risk of hemorrhage, the "retrograde pressure cooker" technique described by Chapot and colleagues should be considered.[45,46] This technique promotes retrograde filling of small-caliber arterial feeders to the shunt leading to complete angiographic obliteration (**Fig. 4**).[20]

In patients who develop sinus stenosis, venous sinus stenting has been proposed as an adjunctive intervention to improve venous outflow. We have

Table 3
Bicêtre neonatal evaluation score

Points	Cardiac	Cerebral	Respiratory	Hepatic	Renal
5	Normal	Normal	Normal	-	-
4	Overload, no medical treatment	Subclinical, isolated EEG abnormalities	Tachypnea, finishes bottle	-	-
3	Failure stabilized with medical treatment	Nonconvulsive clinical neurologic signs	Tachypnea, does not finish bottle	No hepatomegaly, normal function	Normal
2	Failure not stabilized with medical treatment	Isolated convulsions	Assisted ventilation with $Fio_2 < 25\%$	Hepatomegaly, normal function	Transient anuria
1	Ventilation needed	Seizures	Assisted ventilation with $Fio_2 > 25\%$	Moderate or transient hepatic insufficiency	Unstable diuresis with treatment
0	Refractory to medical therapy	Permanent neurologic deficits	Assisted ventilation, desaturations	Abnormal coagulation and elevated LFTs	Anuria

Abbreviations: LFTS, liver function tests.
Maximal score: 21 = 5 (cardiac) + 5 (cerebral) + 5 (respiratory) + 3 (hepatic) + 3 (renal).

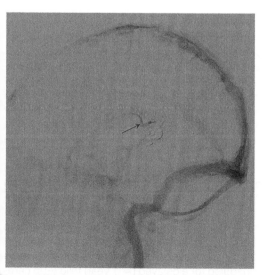

Fig. 2. Subtracted lateral view of the left vertebral artery in late venous phase shows ICV stasis (*red arrow*) concerning for occlusion after obliteration of the VOGM by TVE with pressure cooker technique. A second control run was performed 45 minutes later which demonstrated improved flow through the venous system. The patient returned 6 days later with new acute-onset obstructive hydrocephalus necessitating endoscopic third ventriculostomy.

utilized this in our practice for patients with comorbid posterior fossa sinus stenosis leading to cortical venous congestion and neurologic symptoms with good clinical outcomes without complication.[19]

An early-stage clinical trial has begun to explore the feasibility and utility of in utero partial embolization of the venous pouch for management of patients considered high-risk for neonatal heart failure, as a method to prevent in utero damage and nonviability or multiorgan failure at birth.[47]

ADJUNCTIVE NEUROSURGICAL INTERVENTIONS

There is no role for open neurosurgical intervention currently in primary management of VOGM. Neurosurgical interventions are indicated for the management of hydrocephalus, intracerebral hemorrhage (ICH), or intraventricular hemorrhage (IVH) secondary to the VOGM. VOGM can present with acute or subacute obstructive hydrocephalus due to physical obstruction of the aqueduct by the malformation and chronic nonobstructive hydrocephalus due to reduced cerebrospinal fluid (CSF) absorption secondary to venous congestion.[17,48] To avoid the placement and long-term management of shunt hardware, an endoscopic third ventriculostomy provides a quick relief of acute or subacute hydrocephalus when it can be performed safely.[49] The use of ventriculoperitoneal shunts (VPSs) for CSF

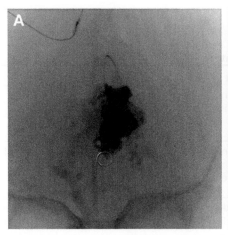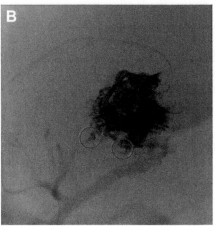

Fig. 3. Subtracted AP (*A*) and lateral (*B*) views of the right internal carotid artery after transarterial embolization from a right pericallosal artery feeder demonstrate devascularization of the left-sided and medial angiogenic network. The EVOH injection was performed to penetrate the network until retrograde filling was noted toward eloquent thalamoperforating feeders in the brainstem (*red circles*).

diversion carries a high rate of complication and should be used as a last resort.[50] In patients who present with slowly developing hydrocephalus, VPS should only be utilized in patients who are poor candidates for embolization or who have maximized endovascular management.

Radiosurgery is rarely utilized as a second-line approach for the obliteration of VOGM. Targeting of the malformation may be challenging especially in VOGM with a high degree of angiogenesis.[22] Radiosurgery does not offer any immediate relief in managing critically unstable VOGM patients, leading to a continued risk of hemorrhage, and

exposes the maturing brain to high levels of radiation.[51] With the improvement of embolization in achieving near or complete VOGM closure, radiosurgery focused on a small remaining malformation may be considered as a means to achieve cure in older children.

CLINICAL FOLLOW-UP AND LONG-TERM CARE

Close follow-up is critical while patients undergo staged embolization. Ischemic strokes, acute-onset new or exacerbation of hydrocephalus, and new-onset seizures may occur between sessions. Establishing a neurologic baseline and tracking the patient's developmental milestones are critical in clinical follow-up to assess for new or worsening symptoms. Embolization sessions should be scheduled 2 to 6 months apart, which includes postprocedural clinic visits to assess the patient's status. Tight follow-up is critical to prevent further development of the VOGM, which can worsen symptoms and significantly complicate future transarterial access with the development of angiogenesis, dural arteriovenous shunts, or venous occlusion or stenosis.[52]

After successful obliteration, patients should be scheduled for a delayed ($\approx$ 1 year) follow-up cerebral angiogram to confirm stable occlusion of the malformation. At this 1 year angiogram, we have seen development of remote dural fistulas.[21] Small residual VOGM may spontaneously completely thrombose between sessions and be seen on angiogram before planned embolization. In these patients, a follow-up angiogram should be offered to confirm stable occlusion.

Fig. 4. A lateral radiograph of the VOGM demonstrates 3 microcatheters in place within the vein of Galen during transvenous embolization by pressure cooker technique.

Table 4
Current molecular markers of vein of Galen malformation and evidence

Broad Function of Gene	Gene	Function and Evidence
Arteriovenous specification genes	EFNB2	Guidance factor for arterial development. Dysregulation of the EphrinB2:EphB4 ratio drives endothelial cell dysfunction in pediatric cerebrovascular AVMs.[58] The EFNB2-EPHB4-RASA1 cassette is a highly implicated marker in VOGM.
	EPHB4	Mutation in CM-AVM2 syndrome. Guidance factor for venous development involved in Ras signaling.[54] Genome-wide burden of damaging heterozygous mutations in a study of 55 probands.[59] Incomplete penetrance of damaging variants.[6]
	NOTCH1	Balanced against EphrinB2:EphB4 ratio in arteriovenous specification. Variants involved in congenital heart defects. Damaging variants identified in integrated WES and single-cell transcriptomics of 310 VOGM proband-family trios.[6]
TGFβ superfamily HHT genes	ACVRL1	Encodes ALK1. Implicated in AD HHT type 2.[56] Rare damaging variant identified in integrated WES and single-cell transcriptomics of 310 trios and multigenerational pedigrees.[6]
	ENG	Encodes endoglin. Implicated in HHT type 2. Identified in isolated VOGM in setting of AD HHT.[55]
VEGFR-Ras signaling of angiogenesis	RASA1	Mutation in CM-AVM1 syndrome.[53] Ubiquitous signal transduction pathway regulating cellular growth and differentiation. Differential expression in fetal cerebral endothelial cells drives angiogenic phenotype.[57] Loss-of-function mutations in integrated WES and single-cell transcriptomics of 310 trios.[6]
	ITGB1	Encodes β1 integrin. Organizes arterial endothelial cell development. Rare damaging variant identified in integrated WES and single-cell transcriptomics of 310 trios.[6]
	PTPN11	Encodes SHP2 which drives vasculogenesis. Rare damaging variant identified in integrated WES and single-cell transcriptomics of 310 trios.[6]

Abbreviations: SHP2, src homology 2-containing protein tyrosine phosphatase 2; TGFb, transforming growth factor beta.
   Note: These genes have significant interplay with each other and have broad, interconnected roles. This is a general categorization of function.

CURRENT AND FUTURE DIRECTIONS FOR VEIN OF GALEN MALFORMATION

Molecular studies of patients with VOGM have begun to elucidate new genomic and proteomic markers linked to the development of VOGM. Isolated VOGMs have historically been described in association with normal Mendelian disorders including autosomal dominant (AD) capillary malformation-AVM (CM-AVM) syndromes with RASA1 and EPHB4 mutations and AD hereditary hemorrhagic telangiectasias (HHTs) with ENG and ACVRL1 mutations.[53–56] However, these were limited to individual cases and used conventional genetic analysis. Greater population-wide success has been seen with the use of whole exome sequencing (WES) to focus on the role of damaging de novo mutations, somatic mosaic presentations, and the incomplete penetrance of rarely transmitted genes suggestive of a 2 hit hypothesis (Table 4). Parents of patients with VOGM have demonstrated various cutaneous vascular malformation phenotypes involving associated mutations.[7] The EFNB2-EPHB4-RASA1 cassette, a mobile genetic element of arteriovenous specification genes, has been heavily implicated along with its downstream signaling pathways. These VOGM genes converge on vascular endothelial growth factor receptor - rat sarcoma virus (VEGFR-Ras) signaling pathways within fetal cerebral endothelial cells, where differential expression of Ras drives proangiogenic or antiangiogenic phenotypes.[57] Studies are being conducted to assess transcriptomic and proteomic changes that lead to the development and regression of angiogenesis linked to VOGM embolization. WES is expected to see increased utility in screening patients and their families to provide genetic counseling and identify eligibility for novel therapeutics.

SUMMARY

Significant efforts have been made over the last few decades to improve the diagnosis, management, and outcomes of patients with VOGM. The mainstays of treatment remain focused on primary endovascular management by staged TAEs with adjunctive use of medical therapy and neurosurgical intervention for symptom control in select patients. A thorough assessment of fetal and postnatal patients with echocardiography and brain MRIs is key to appropriately triaging patients for emergent embolization. Innovation in endovascular technology and transvenous technique now permits greater aggressiveness in endovascular management with high rates of success. Future molecular studies hold significant promise in identifying novel mutations which may serve as therapeutic targets.

CLINICS CARE POINTS

- Antenatal diagnosis of VOGM on normal maternal follow-up visits is critical for timely management decisions.
- Physicians should maintain a low threshold for working up potential VOGM in newborn patients presenting with acute postnatal cardiopulmonary distress if no prenatal imaging was obtained.
- Comprehensive neuroimaging is required to diagnose and evaluate a patient with VOGM.
- Multidisciplinary coordination between cardiology, neonatology, and pediatric neurointervention is necessary to ascertain the need for medical management or early endovascular embolization.
- If indicated, neonatal embolization is used for stabilization of heart failure until patients can later tolerate staged embolizations to reduce and close the shunt.

- Close follow-up is critical to prevent development of intervening angiogenesis between treatment sessions and ensure closure of the shunt.
- Clinic visits should be utilized for long-term neurologic assessment of known VOGM patients and for early diagnosis of infantile VOGM by head circumference growth curves or other symptoms.

REFERENCES

1. Berenstein A, Fifi JT, Niimi Y, et al. Vein of Galen Malformations in Neonates: New Management Paradigms for Improving Outcomes. Yearb Neurol Neurosurg 2012;2012:269–70.
2. Berenstein A, Paramasivam S, Sorscher M, et al. Vein of Galen Aneurysmal Malformation: Advances in Management and Endovascular treatment. Neurosurgery 2019;84(2):469.
3. Lasjaunias PL, Chng SM, Sachet M, et al. The Management of Vein of Galen Aneurysmal Malformations. Neurosurgery 2006;59(suppl_5). S3-S184-S3-194.
4. Recinos PF, Rahmathulla G, Pearl M, et al. Vein of Galen malformations: epidemiology, clinical presentations, management. Neurosurg Clin N Am 2012;23(1):165–77.
5. Lasjaunias P, Berenstein A, ter Brugge KG. Surgical neuroangiography. 2nd edition. New York: Springer Berlin Heidelberg; 2001.
6. Zhao S, Mekbib KY, van der Ent MA, et al. Mutation of key signaling regulators of cerebrovascular development in vein of Galen malformations. Nat Commun 2023;14:7452.
7. Duran D, Karschnia P, Gaillard JR, et al. Human genetics and molecular mechanisms of vein of Galen malformation. J Neurosurg Pediatr 2018;21(4):367–74.
8. Gailloud P, O'Riordan DP, Burger I, et al. Diagnosis and Management of Vein of Galen Aneurysmal Malformations. J Perinatol 2005;25(8):542–51.
9. Khullar D, Andeejani AMI, Bulsara KR. Evolution of treatment options for vein of Galen malformations. J Neurosurg Pediatr 2010;6(5):444–51.
10. Berenstein A, Ortiz R, Niimi Y, et al. Endovascular management of arteriovenous malformations and other intracranial arteriovenous shunts in neonates, infants, and children. Childs Nerv Syst ChNS Off J Int Soc Pediatr Neurosurg 2010;26(10):1345–58.
11. Raybaud C. Normal and Abnormal Embryology and Development of the Intracranial Vascular System. Neurosurg Clin N Am 2010;21(3):399–426.
12. Komiyama M. The median vein of prosencephalon of Markowski: From morphology to genetics. Interv Neuroradiol 2020;26(6):752–6.

13. McElhinney DB, Halbach VV, Silverman NH, et al. Congenital cardiac anomalies with vein of Galen malformations in infants. Arch Dis Child 1998; 78(6):548–51.

14. Friedman AH, Fahey JT. The transition from fetal to neonatal circulation: normal responses and implications for infants with heart disease. Semin Perinatol 1993;17(2):106–21.

15. Patel N, Mills JF, Cheung MMH, et al. Systemic haemodynamics in infants with vein of Galen malformation: assessment and basis for therapy. J Perinatol Off J Calif Perinat Assoc 2007;27(7):460–3.

16. Kehrer M, Blumenstock G, Ehehalt S, et al. Development of cerebral blood flow volume in preterm neonates during the first two weeks of life. Pediatr Res 2005;58(5):927–30.

17. Paramasivam S. Hydrocephalus in Vein of Galen Malformations. Neurol India 2021;69(8):376.

18. Pearl M, Gomez J, Gregg L, et al. Endovascular management of vein of Galen aneurysmal malformations. Influence of the normal venous drainage on the choice of a treatment strategy. Childs Nerv Syst ChNS Off J Int Soc Pediatr Neurosurg 2010; 26(10):1367–79.

19. Berenstein A, Toma N, Niimi Y, et al. Occlusion of Posterior Fossa Dural Sinuses in Vein of Galen Malformation. Am J Neuroradiol 2016;37(6):1092–8.

20. Shigematsu T, Bazil MJ, Fifi JT, et al. Fine, Vascular Network Formation in Patients with Vein of Galen Aneurysmal Malformation. Am J Neuroradiol 2022; 43(10):1481–7.

21. Paramasivam S, Niimi Y, Meila D, et al. Dural Arteriovenous Shunt Development in Patients with Vein of Galen Malformation. Interv Neuroradiol 2014;20(6): 781–90.

22. Buell TJ, Ding D, Starke RM, et al. Embolization-induced angiogenesis in cerebral arteriovenous malformations. J Clin Neurosci Off J Neurosurg Soc Australas 2014;21(11):1866–71.

23. Hansen D, Kan PT, Reddy GD, et al. Pediatric knowledge update: Approach to the management of vein of Galen aneurysmal malformations in neonates. Surg Neurol Int 2016;7(Suppl 12):S317–21.

24. Paladini D, Deloison B, Rossi A, et al. Vein of Galen aneurysmal malformation (VGAM) in the fetus: retrospective analysis of perinatal prognostic indicators in a two-center series of 49 cases. Ultrasound Obstet Gynecol Off J Int Soc Ultrasound Obstet Gynecol 2017;50(2):192–9.

25. Jhaveri S, Berenstein A, Srivastava S, et al. High Output Cardiovascular Physiology and Outcomes in Fetal Diagnosis of Vein of Galen Malformation. Pediatr Cardiol 2021;42(6):1416–24.

26. Schwarz S, Brevis Nuñez F, Dürr NR, et al. Aortic Steal Correlates with Acute Organ Dysfunction and Short-Term Outcomes in Neonates with Vein of Galen Malformation. Neonatology 2023;1–10.

27. Doctor P, Ramaciotti C, Angelis D, et al. Echocardiography evaluation of neonatal vein of Galen aneurysmal malformation. Cardiol Young 2023;1–6.

28. Arko L, Lambrych M, Montaser A, et al. Fetal and Neonatal MRI Predictors of Aggressive Early Clinical Course in Vein of Galen Malformation. Am J Neuroradiol 2020;41(6):1105–11.

29. Cory MJ, Durand P, Sillero R, et al. Vein of Galen aneurysmal malformation: rationalizing medical management of neonatal heart failure. Pediatr Res 2023;93(1):39–48.

30. Schwarz S, Brevis Nuñez F, Dürr NR, et al. Doppler Ultrasound Flow Reversal in the Superior Sagittal Sinus to Detect Cerebral Venous Congestion in Vein of Galen Malformation. AJNR Am J Neuroradiol 2023; 44(6):707–15.

31. D'Amico A, Tinari S, D'Antonio F, et al. Outcome of fetal Vein Galen aneurysmal malformations: a systematic review and meta-analysis. J Matern Fetal Neonatal Med 2022;35(25):5312–7.

32. Jaimes C, Machado-Rivas F, Chen K, et al. Brain Injury in Fetuses with Vein of Galen Malformation and Nongalenic Arteriovenous Fistulas: Static Snapshot or a Portent of More? AJNR Am J Neuroradiol 2022;43(7):1036–41.

33. Hamidi H, Rasouly N, Sadiqi J, et al. CT Features of Galen Vein Aneurysm. Mathews J Case Rep 2016;1(4):1–3.

34. Khurana J, Orbach DB, Gauvreau K, et al. Pulmonary Hypertension in Infants and Children with Vein of Galen Malformation and Association with Clinical Outcomes. J Pediatr 2023;258:113404.

35. EL-Khuffash A, McNamara PJ, Breatnach C, et al. The use of milrinone in neonates with persistent pulmonary hypertension of the newborn - a randomised controlled trial pilot study (MINT 1). J Perinatol 2023; 43(2):168–73.

36. Chakkarapani AA, Gupta S, Jamil A, et al. Effects of inhaled nitric oxide (iNO) in pulmonary hypertension secondary to arteriovenous malformations: a retrospective cohort study from the European iNO registry. Eur J Pediatr 2022;181(11):3915–22.

37. Karam O, da Cruz E, Rimensberger PC. VGAM induced high-flow congestive heart failure responsive to PGE1 infusion. Int J Cardiol 2009;132(2): e60–2.

38. Falsaperla R, Vitaliti G, Mauceri L, et al. Levetiracetam in Neonatal Seizures as First-line Treatment: A Prospective Study. J Pediatr Neurosci 2017;12(1): 24–8.

39. Spiotta AM, James RF, Lowe SR, et al. Balloon-augmented Onyx embolization of cerebral arteriovenous malformations using a dual-lumen balloon: a multicenter experience. J Neurointerventional Surg 2015;7(10):721–7.

40. Ullman H, Jones J, Kaneko N, et al. Flow-directed micro-catheterisation technique over a detachable coil. BMJ Case Rep 2019;12(9):e231549.

41. Baranoski JF, Catapano JS, Albuquerque FC, et al. Rapid ventricular overdrive pacing and other advanced flow-control techniques for the endovascular embolization of vein of Galen malformations. Front Pediatr 2023;11.

42. Altschul D, Paramasivam S, Ortega-Gutierrez S, et al. Safety and efficacy using a detachable tip microcatheter in the embolization of pediatric arteriovenous malformations. Childs Nerv Syst 2014; 30(6):1099–107.

43. Meila D, Hannak R, Feldkamp A, et al. Vein of Galen aneurysmal malformation: combined transvenous and transarterial method using a "kissing microcatheter technique.". Neuroradiology 2012;54(1):51–9.

44. Devarajan A, Schupper AJ, Rossitto CP, et al. Use of a mini balloon microcatheter to facilitate penetration of fine vascular networks and curative embolization in vein of Galen malformations. J Neurointerventional Surg 2023. jnis-2023-020577.

45. Fifi JT, Bazil MJ, Matsoukas S, et al. Evolution of transvenous embolization in vein of Galen malformation: case series and review of the literature. J Neurointerventional Surg 2023;15:579–83.

46. Chapot R, Stracke P, Velasco A, et al. The Pressure Cooker Technique for the treatment of brain AVMs. J Neuroradiol 2014;41(1):87–91.

47. Orbach DB, Wilkins-Haug LE, Benson CB, et al. Transuterine Ultrasound-Guided Fetal Embolization of Vein of Galen Malformation, Eliminating Postnatal Pathophysiology. Stroke 2023;54(6):e231–2.

48. Mortazavi MM, Griessenauer CJ, Foreman P, et al. Vein of Galen aneurysmal malformations: critical analysis of the literature with proposal of a new classification system. J Neurosurg Pediatr 2013;12(3): 293–306.

49. Guil-Ibáñez JJ, García-Pérez F, Gomar-Alba M, et al. ETV as treatment for obstructive hydrocephalus in an aneurysmal malformation of the vein of Galen in infants: case report and review of literature. Childs Nerv Syst ChNS Off J Int Soc Pediatr Neurosurg 2023;39(6):1667–72.

50. Meila D, Grieb D, Melber K, et al. Hydrocephalus in vein of Galen malformation: etiologies and therapeutic management implications. Acta Neurochir 2016;158(7):1279–84.

51. Hosmann A, El-Garci A, Gatterbauer B, et al. Multimodality Management of Vein of Galen Malformations–An Institutional Experience. World Neurosurg 2018;112:e837–47.

52. Meila D, Schmidt C, Melber K, et al. Delayed and incomplete treatment may result in dural fistula development in children with Vein of Galen malformation. Interv Neuroradiol J Peritherapeutic Neuroradiol Surg Proced Relat Neurosci 2018;24(1):82–7.

53. Revencu N, Boon LM, Mendola A, et al. RASA1 mutations and associated phenotypes in 68 families with capillary malformation-arteriovenous malformation. Hum Mutat 2013;34(12):1632–41.

54. Amyere M, Revencu N, Helaers R, et al. Germline Loss-of-Function Mutations in EPHB4 Cause a Second Form of Capillary Malformation-Arteriovenous Malformation (CM-AVM2) Deregulating RAS-MAPK Signaling. Circulation 2017;136(11):1037–48.

55. Tsutsumi Y, Kosaki R, Itoh Y, et al. Vein of Galen aneurysmal malformation associated with an endoglin gene mutation. Pediatrics 2011;128(5):e1307–10.

56. Chida A, Shintani M, Wakamatsu H, et al. ACVRL1 gene variant in a patient with vein of Galen aneurysmal malformation. J Pediatr Genet 2013;2(4): 181–9.

57. Zeng X, Hunt A, Chih Jin S, et al. EphrinB2-EphB4-RASA1 signaling in human cerebrovascular development and disease. Trends Mol Med 2019;25(4): 265–86.

58. Fehnel KP, Penn DL, Duggins-Warf M, et al. Dysregulation of the EphrinB2–EphB4 ratio in pediatric cerebral arteriovenous malformations is associated with endothelial cell dysfunction in vitro and functions as a novel noninvasive biomarker in patients. Exp Mol Med 2020;52(4):658–71.

59. Duran D, Zeng X, Jin SC, et al. Mutations in Chromatin Modifier and Ephrin Signaling Genes in Vein of Galen Malformation. Neuron 2019;101(3):429–43.e4.

Venous Sinus Stent to Treat Paralysis

Kurt Yaeger, MD[a],*, J. Mocco, MD, MS[b]

KEYWORDS

- Brain–computer interface • Neural prosthesis • Paralysis • Stentrode • Superior sagittal sinus

KEY POINTS

- The Stentrode was designed for the transvenous detection of neural activity around the brain motor cortex.
- Preclinical animal studies demonstrated high safety parameters and equivalent effectiveness for transvenous neural recording, compared with traditional epidural and subdural electrodes.
- Initial human results observed that patients with Stentrode can accurately click on a computer screen when paired with eye-tracking technology. Importantly, there were no serious device-related adverse events observed.
- Further clinical studies are ongoing to document the safety and efficacy of the Stentrode in other patient populations.

BACKGROUND

The ability of the human mind to connect with machines has long been in the realm of science fiction. In its simplest form, a brain–computer interface (BCI) is a system that acquires an electrical signal from neuronal activity in the brain, analyzes and interprets it, and sends in response, an electrical or mechanical output. In its earliest stages decades ago, BCI technology used noninvasive, scalp-based electroencephalogram (EEG) to interpret neuronal patterns.[1] However, as higher integrity electrical signals have been required for more advanced outputs, electrodes placed directly on the brain surface (electrocorticography; ECoG) or penetrating depth electrodes inserted into subcortical spaces have been used to enhance the spatial and temporal resolution of neuronal activity.[2] Now, as BCI technology surges in popularity for both medical and scientific purposes, novel technologies are being developed and refined to increase sensitivity, effectiveness, and safety. In this article, we review one such novel technology, Stentrode (Synchron, Inc, New York, USA).

THE BURDEN OF PARALYSIS

Motor paralysis can affect patients with a wide range of neurologic pathologies, ranging from traumatic brain or spine injury, stroke, and neurodegenerative conditions such as amyotrophic lateral sclerosis (ALS). More than 5 million patients in the United States have paralysis that limits their ability to function normally.[3] Paralysis contributes to a high burden of disease, both due to direct factors such as impact on independent activities of daily living (IADLs) and indirect costs such as reliance on a caregiver and inability to work.[4] It is projected that paralysis from stroke alone will increase in the coming decades, with disability-adjusted life years increasing by 50% from 2020 to 2050.[5] While efforts to enhance stroke surveillance and prevention are ongoing, as increasing numbers of patients with paralysis enter acute care, more solutions are needed to aid in their recovery.

a Department of Neurological Surgery, Houston Methodist Hospital, 6560 Fannin Street, Suite 944, Houston, TX 77030, USA; b Department of Neurological Surgery, Mount Sinai Hospital, 1 Gustave Levy Place, New York, NY 10029, USA
* Corresponding author.
E-mail address: kyaeger@houstonmethodist.org

Neurosurg Clin N Am 35 (2024) 375–378
https://doi.org/10.1016/j.nec.2024.03.003

The Stentrode

The Stentrode is a neural interface designed to be deployed within the superior sagittal sinus near the motor cortex. The device includes 16 platinum disc electrodes attached to a self-expanding nitinol stent attached to a trailing wire, which is inserted in a transjugular fashion and connected to an implantable receiver transmitter unit (IRTU).[6] This unit is implanted in an infraclavicular pocket, and external communication is maintained with a computer system via an external telemetry unit. The goal of the Stentrode is to acquire high-fidelity motor cortical electrical activity directly from the bilateral precentral gyri. Given its implantation directly into the cerebral venous sinus, the proposed benefit of the technology is to prevent inflammation, gliosis, and disruption of the blood–brain barrier, as occurs with typical transcranial electrode technologies.[7] During the implantation procedure, a preoperative MRI is fused with the 3-dimensional cerebral angiogram, and target markers are created to aid in deployment in the superior sagittal sinus adjacent to the motor cortex.

INITIAL SCIENTIFIC BASIS FOR TRANSVENOUS BRAIN–COMPUTER INTERFACE

In 2016, the Stentrode developers (Synchron, Inc) published their initial results on the transvascular recording of neural activity in sheep.[8] For this study, the Stentrode device was deployed into the superior sagittal sinus, adjacent to the precentral gyrus. To assess vessel wall incorporation due to endothelialization, Stentrode strut to lumen distance was measured using x-ray imaging between the first day postimplantation and up to 4 months. The devices were found to increase in diameter up to 320 μm at the last follow-up, suggestive of incorporation into the wall of the sagittal sinus. The authors also assessed changes to tissue impedance postimplantation, which showed capacitive increases up to day 28, but maximal effects occurring by day 6. Lastly, the group assessed their endovascular electrocorticography using somatosensory evoked potentials (SSEPs), more specifically the phase reversal of SSEP peak amplitudes, corresponding to the location of the central sulcus. They observed an increased number of electrodes recoding neural activity over time, without any changes in amplitudes, and concluded that a spatial resolution of 2.4 mm was possible using the Stentrode. Overall, the spectral content and bandwidth of the neural activity recorded by the Stentrode were comparable to those of epidural electrodes, but somewhat decreased when compared with subdural electrodes. However, a follow-up study demonstrated equivalent quality of neural recordings between endovascular, subdural, and epidural electrode arrays.[9]

Long-term assessment of Stentrode devices was performed at 190 days to assess the chronic viability of the implants. The neural activity bandwidth remained stable for more than 20 weeks postimplant. While the superior sagittal sinus remained patent in all sheep assessed by cerebral angiogram, there was a reduction in the number of veins draining into the sinus on long-term follow-up. However, this did not correlate with any neurologic sequela. The authors concluded that the transvenous route for neural interface implantation was safe and effective for the chronic recording of neurologic activity.

In 2018, the Synchron authors presented their results on the focal stimulation of the motor cortex in sheep using the Stentrode implanted in the superior sagittal sinus.[10] After implantation, the authors observed facial and limb muscle response to the stimulation of the Stentrode. Furthermore, they concluded that the biggest factor in stimulating a motor response was proximity to the motor cortex, rather than the orientation of the stent in the superior sagittal sinus.

HUMAN TRIALS FOR TRANSVENOUS BRAIN–COMPUTER INTERFACE

Based on the results from animal trials, the Synchron group began a first in human study in Australia (The Stentrode With Thought Controlled Digital Switch/SWITCH trial). The inclusion criteria for the study were patients with a diagnosis of paralysis due to spinal cord injury, ALS, stroke, or muscular dystrophy. All patients needed to have the diagnosis for at least 6 months (≥12 months for spinal cord injury), and evidence of motor cortical activation on functional MRI was required. Patients with dementia or other cognitive or psychiatric conditions were excluded. Patients on chronic immunosuppressant medications or those with incompatible cerebral venous anatomy were also excluded.

In October 2020, the results from the first 2 human subjects were published.[6] For the human trial, the Stentrode was implanted in the superior sagittal sinus adjacent to the precentral gyrus. After implantation and time for incisional healing, a training period began using a battery of tasks associated with motor cortex mapping. A machine-learning decoder was used to couple spectral features of neural activity with specific, predefined movements. An eye-tracking device was used to move a computer mouse cursor. The subjects were trained on 3 possible actions: no click, short click, or long click. Once training was completed, with 90% accuracy on click selection, the subjects were assessed for performance. Both patients achieved click selection accuracy of 93% while typing words on a virtual keyboard, and both were able to carry out everyday activities such as texting, personal finance, and online shopping. Neither patient experienced an adverse event, either intraoperatively or in the follow-up period.

The results from the first 5 patients with Stentrode of the SWITCH trial were published in January 2023.[11] The cohort consisted of 4 patients with ALS, with severe upper extremity paralysis and varying degrees of lung function impairment and speech dysfunction. Regarding safety endpoints, there were no serious device-related adverse events documented in the study. Two patients died due to complications from ALS, unrelated to the device. There were no thromboses or occlusions of the superior sagittal sinus observed on routine follow-up imaging, nor was there any evidence of device migration within the sinus. Regarding the efficacy of the device, neural activity remained strong with high bandwidth throughout the study. After training sessions, all patients were able to use the BCI system at home (with the help of a caregiver) to perform everyday tasks such as texting, emailing, online shopping, and personal finance. Overall, the authors concluded that transvenous BCI has an acceptable safety and efficacy profile when using the Stentrode device, and these studies have shown further proof of concept for endovascular neural recording in humans.

DISCUSSION

Endovascular brain–computer interface (BCI) represents a paradigm shift in the treatment of paralysis. Until recently, human studies in BCI have required patients to undergo invasive surgery with burr holes or craniotomy to obtain high-quality electrical neural recordings. Using a transvenous route to deploy electrodes in the superior sagittal sinus is a novel concept in BCI techniques. Based on the evidence published by the Synchron group, the Stentrode represents a safe and feasible method of allowing patients with paralysis to engage in daily activities.

While the Stentrode is a novel technology, there is a safety precedent for deploying cerebral venous sinus stents in patients with idiopathic intracranial hypertension. In one meta-analysis of 24 studies (473 patients with IIH undergoing venous stenting), the rate of major neurologic complications (such as intracranial hemorrhage or an ischemic event) was 2%.[12] Stentrode implantation requires patients to be on dual antiplatelets for 3 months, with aspirin monotherapy to continue for at least 1 year.

Overall, the Stentrode BCI appears comparable to other invasive BCI technologies, in regard to spatial and temporal resolution as well as training system uptake.[13] Further research will need to be performed to better understand the long-term efficacy and safety of the Stentrode implant.

TECHNOLOGICAL LIMITATIONS

The transvenous BCI system certainly has limitations in its current form. At present, it relies on eye-tracking technology to move a cursor for patients with paralysis. This may not be feasible for many patients. The human studies so far have assessed patients with ALS, and unfortunately many of these patients have serious health conditions that may preclude their participation in long-term follow-up. The requirement for antiplatelet therapy also may complicate these patients' courses. Certainly, more research needs to be performed to advance the technology and make it available to more patient cohorts with paralysis.

SUMMARY

The Stentrode BCI is the first of its kind: a transvenous electrode deployed in the cerebral vasculature to record neural activity. The initial human trials are encouraging and suggest a good safety profile and efficacy in detecting and decoding neural signals. Future human studies are warranted to observe the long-term effects of transvenous BCI for paralysis.

CLINICS CARE POINTS

- The Stentrode was designed for the transvenous detection of neural activity around the brain motor cortex.

- Preclinical animal studies demonstrated high safety parameters and equivalent effectiveness for transvenous neural recording, compared with traditional epidural and subdural electrodes.

- Initial human results observed that patients with Stentrode can accurately click on a computer screen when paired with eye-tracking technology. Importantly, there were no serious device-related adverse events observed.

- Further clinical studies are ongoing to document the safety and efficacy of the Stentrode in other patient populations.

DISCLOSURE

K. Yaeger has no relevant disclosures. J. Mocco is Chief Medical Officer for Synchron a company developing a transvenous BCI for paralysis therapy and therefore has stock and a consulting agreement.

REFERENCES

1. Kawala-Sterniuk A, Browarska N, Al-Bakri A, et al. Summary of over fifty years with brain-computer interfaces—a review. Brain Sci 2021;11(1):1–41.

2. Martini ML, Oermann EK, Opie NL, et al. Sensor modalities for brain-computer interface technology: a comprehensive literature review. Neurosurgery 2020;86(2):E108–17.

3. Armour BS, Courtney-Long EA, Fox MH, et al. Prevalence and causes of paralysis-United States, 2013. Am J Publ Health 2016;106(10):1855–7.

4. Blanes L, Carmagnani MIS, Ferreira LM. Health-related quality of life of primary caregivers of persons with paraplegia. Spinal Cord 2007;45(6): 399–403.

5. Feigin VL, Owolabi MO, Owolabi MO, et al. Pragmatic solutions to reduce the global burden of stroke: a World Stroke Organization-Lancet Neurology Commission. Lancet Neurol 2023;22(12):1160–206.

6. Oxley TJ, Yoo PE, Rind GS, et al. Motor neuroprosthesis implanted with neurointerventional surgery improves capacity for activities of daily living tasks in severe paralysis: first in-human experience. J Neurointerventional Surg 2021;13(2):102–8.

7. Karumbaiah L, Saxena T, Carlson D, et al. Relationship between intracortical electrode design and chronic recording function. Biomaterials 2013; 34(33):8061–74.

8. Oxley TJ, Opie NL, John SE, et al. Minimally invasive endovascular stent-electrode array for high-fidelity, chronic recordings of cortical neural activity. Nat Biotechnol 2016;34(3):320–7.

9. John SE, Opie NL, Wong YT, et al. Signal quality of simultaneously recorded endovascular, subdural and epidural signals are comparable. Sci Rep 2018; 8(1). https://doi.org/10.1038/S41598-018-26457-7.

10. Opie NL, John SE, Rind GS, et al. Focal stimulation of the sheep motor cortex with a chronically implanted minimally invasive electrode array mounted on an endovascular stent. Nat Biomed Eng 2018; 2(12):907–14.

11. Mitchell P, Lee SCM, Yoo PE, et al. Assessment of safety of a fully implanted endovascular brain-computer interface for severe paralysis in 4 patients: the stentrode with thought-controlled digital switch (SWITCH) study. JAMA Neurol 2023;80(3):270–8.

12. Saber H, Lewis W, Sadeghi M, et al. Stent survival and stent-adjacent stenosis rates following venous sinus stenting for idiopathic intracranial hypertension: a systematic review and meta-analysis. Interv Neurol 2018;7(6):490–500.

13. Nuyujukian P, Albites Sanabria J, Saab J, et al. Cortical control of a tablet computer by people with paralysis. PLoS One 2018;13(11). https://doi.org/10.1371/JOURNAL.PONE.0204566.

Endovascular Shunting for Communicating Hydrocephalus Using a Biologically Inspired Transdural Cerebrospinal Fluid Valved eShunt® Implant

Adel M. Malek, MD, PhD[a,b,]*, Brandon M. Beneduce, BS[b],
Carl B. Heilman, MD[a]

KEYWORDS

- Endovascular shunting • Hydrocephalus • Cerebrospinal fluid • eShunt® Implant
- Arachnoid granulations

KEY POINTS

- A transvenous trans-dural approach to communicating hydrocephalus was developed which mimics the function of the arachnoid granulation by shunting CSF to the jugular vein.
- The low profile eShunt implant is delivered using endovascular method percutaneously via the femoral vein and the inferior petrosal sinus into the cerebello-pontine angle cistern.
- Unlike conventional surgical ventriculo-peritoneal or -atrial shunts, the eShunt approach avoids hydrostatic pressure gradient-related siphon effect and may have a reduced rate of infection.
- Preliminary clinical evidence with the eShunt has demonstrated swift reduction of elevated intracranial pressure, leading to initiation of ongoing pilot clinical trials.

INTRODUCTION

Cerebrospinal fluid (CSF) circulation has traditionally been viewed as a bulk-flow process originating from production in choroid plexus of the cerebral ventricles, traveling through the subarachnoid spaces (SASs), up along the cerebral convexities until eventual re-absorption into cerebral venous blood flow.[1] The arachnoid granulations that straddle the dura mater and protrude into the dural venous sinuses, commonly along the superior sagittal sinus, are largely responsible for CSF outflow.[2] Recent work has explored alternative physiologic mechanisms for both CSF production through capillary walls[3] and CSF absorption through extracranial lymphatics,[4] such as the route along the olfactory nerve at the cribiform plate.[5] Nevertheless, the prevailing model describes CSF absorption as a pressure-driven process that occurs through cells of the arachnoid granulations via a natural positive pressure gradient of approximately 3 to 5 mm Hg from the CSF to venous compartments.[2,6] This positive pressure gradient facilitates absorption of CSF from the SAS into the venous system[7–9]; though the magnitude of the pressure gradient can be significantly higher in untreated patients with

[a] Department of Neurosurgery, Tufts Medical Center, 800 Washington Street, Proger 7, Boston, MA 02111, USA; [b] CereVasc Inc., 100 1st Avenue, Bldg. 39, Suite 403, Charlestown Navy Yard, Charlestown, MA 02129, USA
* Corresponding author. Department of Neurosurgery, Tufts Medical Center, 800 Washington Street, Proger 7, Boston, MA 02111.
E-mail address: adel.malek@tuftsmedicine.org

Neurosurg Clin N Am 35 (2024) 379–387
https://doi.org/10.1016/j.nec.2024.03.004
1042-3680/24/© 2024 Elsevier Inc. All rights are reserved, including those for text and data mining, AI training, and similar technologies.

hydrocephalus, typically necessitating surgical intervention for drainage of excess CSF. This concept is witnessed in cases of idiopathic intracranial hypertension where downstream venous sinus stenosis results in upstream venous hypertension impairing CSF absorption through the arachnoid granulations leading to increased CSF pressure.[10] Cerebral venous drainage is known to strongly influence intracranial pressure (ICP), suggesting a regulative mechanism of the venous system over CSF outflow pathways.[11] Lalou and colleagues observed a tight coupling of CSF pressure and sagittal sinus pressure in 10 patients with idiopathic intracranial hypertension using direct measurements through lumbar CSF infusion and cerebral venography. They found CSF pressures slightly exceeding sagittal sinus pressures by a mean 2.34 mm Hg differential and an excellent dynamic correlation (R = 0.96) between the two.[12] The tight coupling of CSF and venous pressures causing them to typically rise and fall in concert helps maintain the positive pressure gradient across the dura in nearly all instances.

When CSF circulation is disrupted, hydrocephalus of either the obstructive or communicating nature may occur. Obstructive hydrocephalus results from a physical blockage along the CSF bulk flow pathway due to structural abnormalities such as tumors, cysts, or congenital malformations. Obstructive hydrocephalus is more common in the pediatric population, often due to congenital malformations such as aqueductal stenosis and constitutes 20% to 30% of all cases. In the greater proportion of cases (60%–70%), communicating hydrocephalus occurs as a result of impaired CSF absorption in the SAS or overproduction of CSF. Communicating hydrocephalus can result from conditions such as subarachnoid hemorrhage, meningitis, traumatic brain injury, or other idiopathic causes, and includes impaired arachnoid granulation function. Communicating hydrocephalus, which will constitute the focus here, is commonly treatable with the placement of a permanent ventricular shunt catheter to divert excess CSF from within the cerebral ventricles to an extracranial compartment such as the peritoneum (ventriculoperitoneal), atrium (ventriculoatrial), or pleural (ventriculopleural) space.

CEREBROSPINAL FLUID SHUNTING

In the United States, the typical shunt configuration for treating communicating hydrocephalus is the ventriculoperitoneal approach,[13] though the ventriculopleural approach is considered in cases of abdominal contraindications. The less common ventriculoatrial route has been shown to exhibit comparable efficacy and safety.[14] The ventriculoatrial approach is regaining interest as the resulting rates of safety and effectiveness have been demonstrated to be similar to the ventriculoperitoneal method.[15]

Although CSF shunting is effective and leads to marked symptom resolution and quality of life improvement,[16] conventional ventricular catheter-based procedures are still accompanied by frequent intra-procedural and post-procedural complications. A 2015 N.I.H.-sponsored symposium titled "Opportunities for Hydrocephalus Research: Pathways to Better Outcomes" noted that "[d]espite many advances in the design of the CSF shunt, there have been few improvements in the rate of shunt malfunction, with greater than 40% of first-time shunts failing within 2 years".[17] A single-institution study conducted at Rigshospitalet in Denmark reported contemporary shunt revision rates of 42.6%, with an average time to first revision of 7.51 months. These findings did not demonstrate a significant decrease when compared to the data from the period 1958 to 1989 (P = .060).[18] The 2017 United Kingdom Shunt Registry database reporting on 3000 annual operations described that 47% of adult and 66.5% of pediatric shunt procedures were revision surgeries to repair or replace failed devices.[19] A 2015 analysis of the US Nationwide Readmissions Database identified a 47.4% reoperation rate in adults within 30 days of index shunt placement and describe that "outcomes of shunt surgery for patients with hydrocephalus treated at unselected institutions are substantially worse than what might be expected based on a reading of the existing literature from major research centers."[20] Single-center reports of adult patients with communicating hydrocephalus describe 1 year shunt revision rates of 34%[21] and serious adverse event rates of 40%.[22] Taken together, these reports have motivated the researchers to seek an alternative approach to treatment of communicating hydrocephalus.

ENDOVASCULAR APPROACH

Adopting a biologically inspired approach, we proposed the design of an implantable device equivalent to the arachnoid granulation, that could be implanted using a minimally invasive endovascular technique (U.S. Patent# 11278708B2). Utilizing the natural CSF outflow mechanism of the arachnoid granulations and the closely linked pressures between the CSF and venous compartments, establishing a hydraulic connection between the CSF-filled SAS or cisterns and the adjacent dural venous sinuses may offer a more physiologic approach to drainage in the treatment of communicating hydrocephalus. A novel trans-dural CSF shunt design that aims to mimic the arachnoid granulations was contemplated to maintain a permanent CSF outflow path through the dura using a delivery catheter with a balloon-based stabilizing mechanism within the venous circulation (**Fig. 1**).

Advances in percutaneous neuroendovascular interventions and supporting imaging techniques have become wide-spread over the past 25 years, with ruptured cerebral aneurysms now predomi-nantly treated using endovascular methods[23] rather than microsurgical clipping. More recently, treatment of embolic ischemic stroke is now rec-ommended for emergent revascularization using mechanical thrombectomy because of proven improved clinical outcomes compared to throm-bolytic therapy alone.[24] The expanded role for endovascular neurointervention has increased the availability of high-resolution neuroimaging angiosuites not only at major medical centers but increasingly in smaller hospitals across the United States and worldwide.

A transvenous transfemoral (or transbrachial or transjugular) catheter-based delivery approach was elected for the development of deployment methods for the proposed endovascular CSF shunt (see **Fig. 1**B). The cerebellopontine angle (CPA) cistern was selected as the target deploy-ment location, a capacious CSF-containing SAS at the lateral surface of the pons and the anterior portion of the cerebellum. This cistern resides adjacent the inferior petrosal sinus (IPS), a dural venous sinus traveling along the skull base at the posterior inferior edge of the petrous bone, lateral to the clivus draining the cavernous sinus into the internal jugular vein (**Fig. 2**). The IPS is commonly traversed for neurovascular procedures such embolization of cavernous sinus arteriovenous fis-tulas[25] and venous sinus sampling for the diag-nosis of Cushing's disease.[26] This prompted a formal anatomic analysis of the CPA cistern and adjacent IPS for greater understanding of the crit-ical dimensions to form the basis of engineering development of an endovascular implant and more precise identification of a target deployment site.[27] The notable aspect is the advantageous for-mation of an apex at the junction of the horizontal and vertical segment of the IPS. This geometric feature confers the ability to consistently reach it as a target site with a co-linear force vector allow-ing transdural access with simple translation (straight-shot approach) without the need for a potentially traumatic stabilizing element such as a balloon or stent as initially envisioned (see **Fig. 1**B). The other advantage of the IPS resides

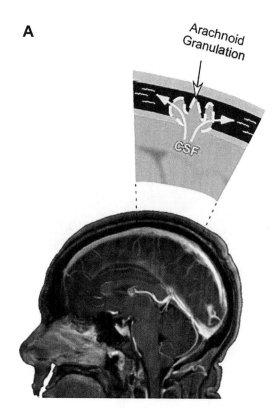

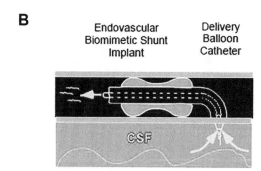

Fig. 1. Arachnoid granulations transdurally straddle the superior sagittal sinus and facilitate physiologic CSF outflow from the subarachnoid space into cere-bral venous drainage (A). The initial innovative concept for the endovascular CSF shunt aimed to replicate this natural process using a biologically inspired transvenously delivered shunt which would be placed within one of the venous sinuses using a stabilizing delivery method possibly involving tran-sient inflation of a nonocclusive balloon to enable transdural advancement of a device into a CSF cistern or space thereby mimicking arachnoid granulation function (B).

in its 270° circumferential bony encasement enabling the controlled advancement of endovas-cular catheters and devices without concern for inducing geometric changes of the underlying

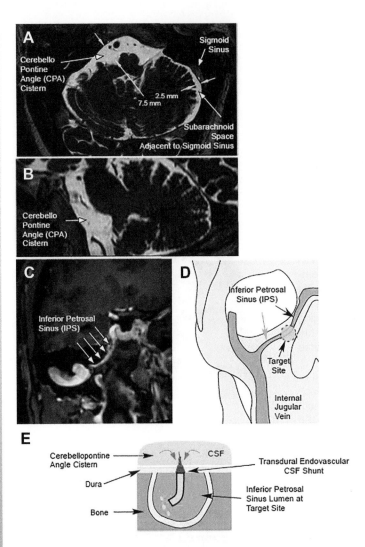

Fig. 2. Exploratory analysis of optimal endovascular shunt transdural delivery location aimed to identify the optimal venous sinus location balancing safety, ease of delivery, and presence of a stable defined CSF reservoir. Axial T2-weighted MRI (*A*) shows proximity of the sigmoid sinus to cerebellar subarachnoid space measuring approximately 2.5 mm in orthogonal depth, compared to the capacious 7.5 mm depth of the cerebellopontine angle cistern (CPA), sagittal view (*B*). T1-weighted gadolinium-enhanced multiplanar reconstruction (*C*) reveals the course of the inferior petrosal sinus (IPS; *arrows*) which lies adjacent to the CPA cistern (separated by dural layer). Target deployment site in the IPS lies at the intersection of the horizontal (green) and vertical (blue) portions of the IPS presenting a reachable inflection angle favoring reproducible device delivery (*D*). Cross-sectional schematic of IPS at target site showing taut dural layer within the channel which is stable mechanically, thanks to circumferential bony confines enabling accurate placement and transdural deployment (*E*).

vessel as is often seen with deployment of intracranial stents or thrombectomy stentrievers. This in turn facilitates sub-millimetric imaging and control using existing roadmapping guidance for the critical step of transdural access into the adjacent CPA cistern.

A low-profile 3.5 cm long biomimetic endovascular shunt (eShunt® Implant; CereVasc, Inc., Charlestown, MA, USA) was developed to straddle the IPS dura at this location featuring a self-expanding malecot at its CSF inflow located in the CPA cistern. The eShunt slender body travels down the IPS leading to a slit-valve-controlled CSF outlet residing in the region of the jugular bulb thus providing a one-way path for excess CSF above a threshold pressure gradient to flow into the venous system (**Fig. 3**A). The device was designed with a smooth, tubular body to encourage maintenance of smooth laminar venous

blood flow around the device and minimize the risk of shear-induced platelet activation and thrombus formation (**Fig. 3**B). A self-expanding malecot protects the inlet from membranous obstruction and prevents IPS venous flow induced distal migration of the implant, thus maintaining a mechanically stable placement within the CPA cistern (**Fig. 3**C). The 3.5 cm length of the device enables it to connect from the CPA cistern through the IPS to its termination within the internal jugular vein in the greatest majority of patient anatomies. In order to enable regulation of CSF outflow, a simple slit valve residing at the implant's venous-end within the internal jugular vein was engineered to open when CSF pressure exceeds venous pressure by a cracking pressure threshold, targeting 10 cc/hour CSF outflow rate in the range of the naturally occurring positive pressure differential of 8 mm Hg or lesser (**Fig. 3**D). This differential pressure valve

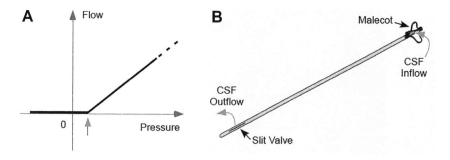

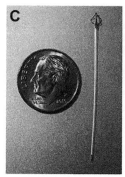
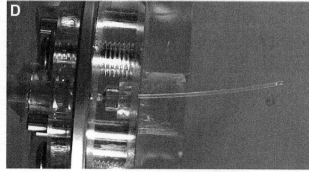

Fig. 3. Idealized pressure-flow characteristics (*A*) for design of the endovascular CSF shunt (eShunt®) enabling forward flow beyond a threshold cracking value (gray *arrow*) and preventing back flow when venous pressures transiently exceed intracranial pressure. Iterative bioengineering processes established the optimal eShunt Implant design (*B*) with a hemocompatible smooth tubular venous end terminated by a differential pressure slit valve, and self-expanding malecot at the inlet-end to maintain stability and prevent migration. Actual eShunt implant next to US dime coin (*C*). Valve testing under normal and supraphysiologic pressure conditions confirmed implant performance (*D*) here showing use of a blue dye for visual assessment of valve function.

design enables fluctuation of the degree of slit opening and self-adjustment of the flow rate according to the dynamic CSF : venous pressure differential, which may vary wIth naturally occurring cyclical waveforms, posture changes, or simple patient to patient variation.

In both healthy and pathologic patients, normal ICP fluctuations occur due to cardiac cycle, respiratory cycle, and other physiologic influences, in addition to gross changes in body positioning.[28] ICP measurements taken from healthy individuals showed that while mean ICP was 11 mm Hg, the range expanded as wide as 8 to 32 mm Hg over a 30 minute recording period, with a pulse wave amplitude of 1 to 3 mm Hg.[29] ICP waveform patterns have been studied extensively and have been found to differ from patient to patient depending on their condition.[30] Patterns can vary from low amplitude and stable average ICP to more irregular waveforms.[31] This natural variability in ICP necessitates a simple valve design that facilitates rather than augments pressure-driven CSF absorption. Thus, the self-regulating

differential pressure valve design is ideally suited for function as an arachnoid granulation surrogate by allowing the appropriate amount of CSF outflow determined by the patient's specific pressure gradient across the implant.

Nevertheless, certain transient physiologic conditions (eg, coughing, straining, sneezing) can cause momentary spikes in venous blood pressure that may exceed ICP, typically occurring for less than 2 seconds.[32–34] The slit valve is designed to close during these conditions when venous pressure meets or exceeds CSF pressure, preventing venous blood reflux through the device and into the SAS.

Unlike ventriculo-peritoneal(VP) shunts, the eShunt Implant is nearly "posture-independent" as the overall implant length does not pose a significant siphoning risk when the patient changes posture from the supine to upright position. Inherent in conventional ventriculoperitoneal or ventriculoatrial shunt designs is a large height difference between the proximal and distal catheter openings in the upright body position that can

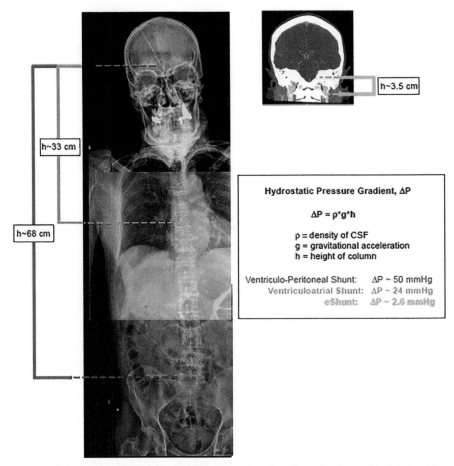

Fig. 4. Illustration of the hydrostatic pressure gradient favoring the eShunt Implant with side-by-side comparison of a ventriculoperitoneal shunt with reconstructed radiographic shunt series (left) illustrating the heights for a ventriculoperitoneal shunt (red) and a ventriculoatrial (orange) compared to the endovascular eShunt CSF shunt implant (right). The short height of the eShunt (~3.5 cm) is associated with a negligible 10–20x smaller hydrostatic pressure gradient seen with patient postural change. Hydrostatic pressure gradient, ΔP $\Delta P = \rho \text{*} g \text{*} h$ ρ = density of CSF. g, gravitational acceleration h, height of column ventriculoperitoneal shunt: ΔP ~50 mm Hg Ventriculoatrial shunt: ΔP ~24 mm Hg eShunt: ΔP ~2.6 mm Hg.

result in large hydrostatic pressure gradients ranging between −18 and −55 mm Hg[35,36] when the patient moves from the supine to upright position. This can result in a siphoning effect during which over-drainage of CSF occurs, reducing ICP to as low as −22 to −32 mm Hg.[36–38] The comparative theoretic magnitude of hydrostatic pressures between a standard CSF shunt and the eShunt Implant are such that the latter's short length of 3.5 cm provides a theoretic 10x or greater reduction of hydrostatic pressures during a postural change, thereby minimizing the risk of overdrainage complications (**Fig. 4**).

Delivery of the eShunt Implant involves a percutaneous transvenous transfemoral procedure and navigation of a delivery catheter into the IPS under fluoroscopic roadmap guidance. This is aided by an imaging workflow based on 3D cone-beam computed tomography venographic reconstruction to highlight the venous anatomy. The resulting 3D volume serves as the basis for 3D-roadmap guidance and for controlled device transdural advancement into the CPA cistern (**Fig. 5**).

CLINICAL IMPLICATIONS

The intended physiologic differential pressure valve is designed for application across a variety of communicating hydrocephalus etiologies. The first pilot clinical study of the eShunt® System (Clinicaltrials.gov #NCT04758611) was initiated in patients with intractable hydrocephalus following aneurysmal subarachnoid hemorrhage. Standard of care management of this patient population involves placement of an external ventricular drain with continuous ICP monitoring capabilities,

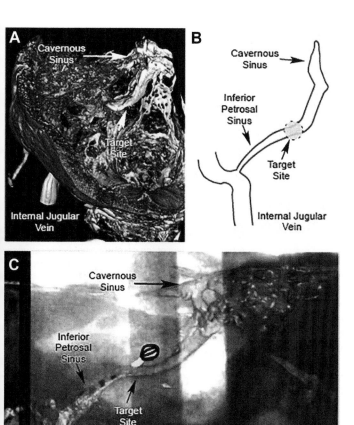

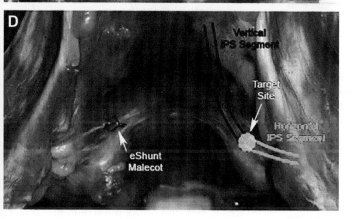

Fig. 5. The anatomy of the bilateral inferior petrosal sinus is well known to the neurovascular practitioner (*A*), with its origin draining the cavernous sinus into the superior aspect of the internal jugular vein. Its fixed position within the petroclival fissure provides a stable platform for traversing the dura in controlled manner to gain access to CSF-filled cerebellopontine angle cistern (*B*). Live fluoroscopic roadmap guidance using 3D overlay technique during the Implant procedure provides high resolution visual feedback during endovascular delivery to confirm cisternal access and accurate implant deployment (*C*). View from top of the skull base in cadaveric specimen showing the eShunt Implant deployed in its target site with its malecot in the CPA cistern (*D*, left) and schematic overlay of the contralateral IPS channel segments (*D*, right).

providing the ability to obtain objective data of eShunt Implant function after placement. Closure of the external ventricular drain prior to the eShunt Procedure enabled real-time evaluation of ICP prior to and following eShunt Implant placement. The first case of an eShunt Implant placement in a patient with this condition resulted in swift reduction of baseline elevated ICP (38 cmH$_2$O) into the normal range (<20 cmH$_2$O) within 90 minutes of implantation.[39] After confirmation of eShunt Implant function via continuous ICP monitoring

over 39 hours postprocedure, which stabilized at approximately 13.5 cmH$_2$O and remained within the normal range, the external ventricular drain was removed. Enrollment of additional patients in this clinical trial remains ongoing.

This successful result of treating communicating hydrocephalus prompted the assessment of the eShunt Implant in patients with normal pressure hydrocephalus. Two prospective, open-label, single-arm pilot studies of the eShunt System commenced in the normal pressure hydrocephalus population in Argentina and the United States (Clinicaltrials.gov #NCT05250505, #NCT05232838) after achieving investigational device exemption from the respective regulatory bodies.

The eShunt Implant may also be useful for the treatment of idiopathic intracranial hypertension, where conventional shunt placement of the ventricular catheter may be complicated by slit ventricles. Stenosis of the transverse or sigmoid sinus present in many of these patients, which may cause venous congestion that contributes to obstruction of CSF outflow and resulting elevated ICP, is upstream from the location of eShunt Implant valve placement.

SUMMARY

The novel endovascular shunting approach was developed to mitigate the common failure modes found with conventional VP shunts such as infection, overdrainage, and obstruction. Neurointerventional procedures have consistently been shown to exhibit infection rates less than 1%.[40,41] The novel implant deployment location and differential pressure-dependent valve design enable self-adjustment of the flow rate according to the dynamic ICP : VBP differential, thereby potentially reducing the risk of drainage complications. Placement in the CPA cistern may mitigate the risk of obstruction typically attributed to choroid plexus ingrowth or contact with ventricular wall ependyma or adjacent white matter.[42] The endovascular delivery method eschews the need to traverse brain parenchyma and white matter in contrast to conventional ventricular catheter-based surgical shunting. Ongoing clinical trials are providing incremental data on the utility, efficacy, and safety of endovascular shunt treatment of differing etiologies of communicating hydrocephalus including post-subarachnoid hemorrhage, and in patients with normal pressure hydrocephalus and idiopathic intracranial hypertension.

DISCLOSURE

Dr. Malek and Heilman are co-inventors of the eShunt® implant, and co-founders of, shareholders in, and consultants for CereVasc Inc.

REFERENCES

1. Brinker T, Stopa E, Morrison J, et al. A new look at cerebrospinal fluid circulation. Fluids Barriers CNS 2014;11(1):10.
2. Pollay M. The function and structure of the cerebrospinal fluid outflow system. Cerebrospinal Fluid Res 2010;7(1):9.
3. Orešković D, Klarica M. The formation of cerebrospinal fluid: Nearly a hundred years of interpretations and misinterpretations. Brain Res Rev 2010;64(2):241–62.
4. Proulx ST. Cerebrospinal fluid outflow: a review of the historical and contemporary evidence for arachnoid villi, perineural routes, and dural lymphatics. Cell Mol Life Sci 2021;78(6):2429–57.
5. Spera I, Cousin N, Ries M, et al. Open pathways for cerebrospinal fluid outflow at the cribriform plate along the olfactory nerves. EBioMedicine 2023;91:104558.
6. Glimcher SA, Holman DW, Lubow M, et al. Ex Vivo Model of Cerebrospinal Fluid Outflow across Human Arachnoid Granulations. Investig Opthalmology Vis Sci 2008;49(11):4721.
7. Spector R, Snodgrass SR, Johanson CE. A balanced view of the cerebrospinal fluid composition and functions: Focus on adult humans. Exp Neurol 2015;273:57–68.
8. Hladky SB, Barrand MA. Mechanisms of fluid movement into, through and out of the brain: evaluation of the evidence. Fluids Barriers CNS 2014;11(1):26.
9. Kapoor KG, Katz SE, Grzybowski DM, et al. Cerebrospinal fluid outflow: An evolving perspective. Brain Res Bull 2008;77(6):327–34.
10. Fargen KM, Coffman S, Torosian T, et al. "Idiopathic" intracranial hypertension: An update from neurointerventional research for clinicians. Cephalalgia 2023;43(4). 03331024231161323.
11. Wilson MH. Monro-Kellie 2.0: The dynamic vascular and venous pathophysiological components of intracranial pressure. J Cereb Blood Flow Metab 2016;36(8):1338–50.
12. Lalou AD, Czosnyka M, Czosnyka ZH, et al. Coupling of CSF and sagittal sinus pressure in adult patients with pseudotumour cerebri. Acta Neurochir 2020;162(5):1001–9.
13. Alvi MA, Brown D, Yolcu Y, et al. Prevalence and trends in management of idiopathic normal pressure hydrocephalus in the United States: insights from the national inpatient sample. World Neurosurg 2021;145:e38–52.
14. Hung AL, Vivas-Buitrago T, Adam A, et al. Ventriculoatrial versus ventriculoperitoneal shunt complications in idiopathic normal pressure hydrocephalus. Clin Neurol Neurosurg 2017;157:1–6.
15. McGovern RA, Kelly KM, Chan AK, et al. Should ventriculoatrial shunting be the procedure of choice for normal-pressure hydrocephalus?: Clinical article. J Neurosurg 2014;120(6):1458–64.
16. Petersen J, Hellström P, Wikkelsø C, et al. Improvement in social function and health-related quality of life after shunt surgery for idiopathic normal-pressure hydrocephalus: Clinical article. J Neurosurg 2014;121(4):776–84.
17. McAllister JP, Williams MA, Walker ML, et al. An update on research priorities in hydrocephalus: overview of the third National Institutes of Health-

sponsored symposium "Opportunities for Hydrocephalus Research: Pathways to Better Outcomes." J Neurosurg 2015;123(6):1427–38.

18. Mansson PK, Johansson S, Ziebell M, et al. Forty years of shunt surgery at Rigshospitalet, Denmark: a retrospective study comparing past and present rates and causes of revision and infection. BMJ Open 2017;7:e013389.

19. Pickard J, Richards H, Seeley H, et al. UK Shunt Registry: Draft Report 2017. 2017. Available at: https://www.brainmic.nihr.ac.uk/wp-content/uploads/2021/12/UKSRDraftReport2017FINAL-min.pdf.

20. LeHanka A, Piatt J. Readmission and reoperation for hydrocephalus: a population-based analysis across the spectrum of age. J Neurosurg 2021;134(4):1210–7.

21. Anderson IA, Saukila LF, Robins JMW, et al. Factors associated with 30-day ventriculoperitoneal shunt failure in pediatric and adult patients. J Neurosurg 2018;130(1):145–53.

22. Kotagal V, Walkowiak E, Heth JA. Serious adverse events following Normal Pressure Hydrocephalus surgery. Clin Neurol Neurosurg 2018;170:113–5.

23. Molyneux AJ, Birks J, Clarke A, et al. The durability of endovascular coiling versus neurosurgical clipping of ruptured cerebral aneurysms: 18 year follow-up of the UK cohort of the International Subarachnoid Aneurysm Trial (ISAT). Lancet 2015;385(9969):691–7.

24. Berkhemer OA, Fransen PSS, Beumer D, et al. A Randomized Trial of Intraarterial Treatment for Acute Ischemic Stroke. N Engl J Med 2015;372(1):11–20.

25. Castro-Afonso LH, Trivelato FP, Rezende MT, et al. The routes for embolization of dural carotid cavernous fistulas when the endovascular approach is indicated as a first-line strategy. Interv Neuroradiol 2018;25(1):66–70.

26. Miller DL, Doppman JL. Petrosal Sinus Sampling: Technique and Rationale. Radiology 1991;178:37–47.

27. Heilman CB, Basil GW, Beneduce BM, et al. Anatomical characterization of the inferior petrosal sinus and adjacent cerebellopontine angle cistern for development of an endovascular transdural cerebrospinal fluid shunt. J Neurointerventional Surg 2019;11(6):598.

28. Eide PK, Sorteberg W. Diagnostic Intracranial Pressure Monitoring and Surgical Management in Idiopathic Normal Pressure Hydrocephalus: A 6-Year

Review of 214 Patients. Neurosurgery 2010;66(1):80–91.

29. Albeck MJ, Børgesen SE, Gjerris F, et al. Intracranial pressure and cerebrospinal fluid outflow conductance in healthy subjects. J Neurosurg 1991;74(4):597–600.

30. Czosnyka M, Czosnyka Z, Keong N, et al. Pulse pressure waveform in hydrocephalus: what it is and what it isn't. Neurosurg Focus 2007;22(4):1–7.

31. Czosnyka M, Pickard JD. Monitoring and interpretation of intracranial pressure. J Neurol Neurosurg Psychiatry 2004;75(6):813.

32. Williams B. Cerebrospinal fluid pressure changes in response to coughing. Brain 1976;99(2):331–46.

33. Little WC, Reeves RC, Coughlan C, et al. Effect of cough on coronary perfusion pressure: Does coughing help clear the coronary arteries of angiographic contrast medium? Circulation 1982;65(3):604–10.

34. Fisher J, Vaghaiwalla F, Tsitlik J, et al. Determinants and clinical significance of jugular venous valve competence. Circulation 1982;65(1):188–96.

35. Pople IK. Hydrocephalus and shunts: what the neurologist should know. J Neurol Neurosurg Psychiatry 2002;73(suppl 1):i17.

36. Czosnyka Z, Czosnyka M, Richards HK, et al. Posture-related overdrainage: comparison of the performance of 10 hydrocephalus shunts in vitro. Neurosurgery 1998;42(2):327–34.

37. Aschoff A, Kremer P, Benesch C, et al. Overdrainage and shunt technology. Child's Nerv Syst 1995;11(4):193–202.

38. Chapman PH, Cosman ER, Arnold MA. The Relationship between Ventricular Fluid Pressure and Body Position in Normal Subjects and Subjects with Shunts: A Telemetric Study. Neurosurgery 1990;26(2):181–9.

39. Lylyk P, Lylyk I, Bleise C, et al. First-in-human endovascular treatment of hydrocephalus with a miniature biomimetic transdural shunt. J Neurointerventional Surg 2022;14(5):495–9.

40. Burkhardt JK, Tanweer O, Litao M, et al. Infection risk in endovascular neurointerventions: a comparative analysis of 549 cases with and without prophylactic antibiotic use. J Neurosurg 2020;132(3):797–801.

41. Kelkar PS, Fleming JB, Walters BC, et al. Infection Risk in Neurointervention and Cerebral Angiography. Neurosurgery 2013;72(3):327–31.

42. Blegvad C, Skjolding AD, Broholm H, et al. Pathophysiology of shunt dysfunction in shunt treated hydrocephalus. Acta Neurochir 2013;155(9):1763–72.

Printed and bound by CPI Group (UK) Ltd, Croydon, CR0 4YY

08/05/2025

01864750-0012